Reaching and Investing in CHILDREN at the MARGINS

Summary of a Joint Workshop
by the National Academies of Sciences, Engineering, and Medicine;
Open Society Foundations; and the International Step by Step
Association (ISSA)

Charlee Alexander, *Rapporteur*

Forum on Investing in Young Children Globally

Board on Global Health

Board on Children, Youth, and Families

Health and Medicine Division

Division of Behavioral and Social Sciences and Education

The National Academies of
SCIENCES · ENGINEERING · MEDICINE

THE NATIONAL ACADEMIES PRESS
Washington, DC
www.nap.edu

THE NATIONAL ACADEMIES PRESS 500 Fifth Street, NW Washington, DC 20001

This activity was supported by grants from Autism Speaks (unnumbered award); the Bernard van Leer Foundation (222-2012-043); The Bill & Melinda Gates Foundation (OPP1084405); the Doris Duke Charitable Foundation; the Fraser Mustard Institute for Human Development; Fundação Maria Cecilia Souto Vidigal (unnumbered); Grand Challenges Canada (unnumbered); HighScope Educational Research Foundation (unnumbered); the Inter-American Development Bank (unnumbered); the Jacobs Foundation (2013-1079); Lumos; the National Institutes of Health—Fogarty International Center, the National Institute of Child Health and Human Development, and the National Institute of Mental Health; Nestlé Nutrition Institute (unnumbered); the Open Society Institute–Budapest Foundation (OR2013-10010); ReadyNation (unnumbered); the Robert Wood Johnson Foundation; the Society for Research in Child Development (unnumbered); UNICEF (unnumbered); U.S. Agency for International Development; U.S. Centers for Disease Control and Prevention; and the World Bank (unnumbered). Any opinions, findings, conclusions, or recommendations expressed in this publication do not necessarily reflect the views of any organization or agency that provided support for the project.

International Standard Book Number-13: 978-0-309-44101-8
International Standard Book Number-10: 0-309-44101-3
Digital Object Identifier: 10.17226/23491

Additional copies of this workshop summary are available for sale from the National Academies Press, 500 Fifth Street, NW, Keck 360, Washington, DC 20001; (800) 624-6242 or (202) 334-3313; http://www.nap.edu.

Printed in the United States of America

Suggested citation: National Academies of Sciences, Engineering, and Medicine. 2016. *Reaching and investing in children at the margins: Summary of a joint workshop.* Washington, DC: The National Academies Press. doi: 10.17226/23491.

The National Academies of
SCIENCES · ENGINEERING · MEDICINE

The **National Academy of Sciences** was established in 1863 by an Act of Congress, signed by President Lincoln, as a private, nongovernmental institution to advise the nation on issues related to science and technology. Members are elected by their peers for outstanding contributions to research. Dr. Ralph J. Cicerone is president.

The **National Academy of Engineering** was established in 1964 under the charter of the National Academy of Sciences to bring the practices of engineering to advising the nation. Members are elected by their peers for extraordinary contributions to engineering. Dr. C. D. Mote, Jr., is president.

The **National Academy of Medicine** (formerly the Institute of Medicine) was established in 1970 under the charter of the National Academy of Sciences to advise the nation on medical and health issues. Members are elected by their peers for distinguished contributions to medicine and health. Dr. Victor J. Dzau is president.

The three Academies work together as the **National Academies of Sciences, Engineering, and Medicine** to provide independent, objective analysis and advice to the nation and conduct other activities to solve complex problems and inform public policy decisions. The Academies also encourage education and research, recognize outstanding contributions to knowledge, and increase public understanding in matters of science, engineering, and medicine.

Learn more about the National Academies of Sciences, Engineering, and Medicine at **www.national-academies.org**.

PLANNING COMMITTEE ON REACHING AND INVESTING IN CHILDREN AT THE MARGINS[1]

LIANA GHENT, Director, International Step by Step Association (ISSA)
JODY HEYMANN, Dean, Fielding School of Public Health, University of California, Los Angeles
GILLIAN HUEBNER, Senior Associate, Maestral International[2]
TINA HYDER, Deputy Director, Early Childhood Program, London, Open Society Foundations
PETRA KACIRKOVA, Country Director, Czech Republic, Lumos Foundation
SARAH KLAUS, Director, Early Childhood Program, London, Open Society Foundations
VESNA KUTLESIC, Director, Office of Global Health, *Eunice Kennedy Shriver* National Institute of Child Health and Human Development, National Institutes of Health
JOAN LOMBARDI, Senior Advisor, Bernard van Leer Foundation
ANN MASTEN, Distinguished McKnight University Professor, Institute of Child Development, University of Minnesota, Minneapolis
SIMON SOMMER, Head of Research, Jacobs Foundation
AMALIA WAXMAN, Consultant

[1] The National Academies of Sciences, Engineering, and Medicine's planning committees are solely responsible for organizing the workshop, identifying topics, and choosing speakers. The responsibility for the published workshop summary rests with the workshop rapporteur and the institution.
[2] Former Policy and Advocacy Director at Lumos Foundation until December 31, 2015.

FORUM ON INVESTING IN YOUNG CHILDREN GLOBALLY[1]

---

[1] The National Academies of Sciences, Engineering, and Medicine's forums and roundtables do not issue, review, or approve individual documents. The responsibility for the published workshop summary rests with the workshop rapporteur and the institution.

[2] Former Colombian National Coordinator of the Intersectoral Commission for Early Childhood, Presidency of the Republic, Colombia, until December 31, 2015.

JODY HEYMANN, Dean, Fielding School of Public Health, University of California, Los Angeles
GILLIAN HUEBNER, Senior Associate, Maestral International[3]
VENITA KAUL, Director, School of Education Studies, and Director, Center for Early Childhood Education and Development, Ambedkar University, Delhi
SARAH KLAUS, Director, Early Childhood Program, London, Open Society Foundations
VESNA KUTLESIC, Director, Office of Global Health, *Eunice Kennedy Shriver* National Institute of Child Health and Human Development, National Institutes of Health
ALBERT LEE, Professor (Clinical), Jockey Club School of Public Health and Primary Care, and Director, Centre for Health, Education, and Health Promotion, Chinese University of Hong Kong
JOAN LOMBARDI, Senior Advisor, Bernard van Leer Foundation
STEPHEN LYE, Executive Director, Fraser Mustard Institute of Human Development, University of Toronto
KOFI MARFO, Professor and Foundation Director, Institute for Human Development, Aga Khan University (South-Central Asia, East Africa, United Kingdom)
MARK MILLER, Director, Division of International and Population Studies, Fogarty International Center, National Institutes of Health
HELIA MOLINA MILMAN, Vice Dean, Research and Development, Faculty of Medical Sciences, University de Santiago de Chile and Former Minister of Health, Chile
ARIEL PABLOS-MÉNDEZ, Assistant Administrator for Global Health, U.S. Agency for International Development
JANNA PATTERSON, Senior Program Officer, Maternal, Newborn and Child Health, The Bill & Melinda Gates Foundation
ALAN PENCE, United Nations Educational, Scientific and Cultural Organization Chair, Early Childhood, Education, Care and Development and Professor, School of Child and Youth Care, University of Victoria
RUTH PEROU, Lead Behavioral Scientist, Office of the Director, National Center on Birth Defects and Developmental Disabilities, U.S. Centers for Disease Control and Prevention
CHERYL POLK, President, HighScope Educational Research Foundation
EDUARDO QUEIROZ, Executive Director, Fundação Maria Cecilia Souto Vidigal
JOSE SAAVEDRA, Global Chief Medical Officer, Nestlé Nutrition

[3] Former Policy and Advocacy Director at Lumos Foundation until December 31, 2015.

LORRAINE SHERR, Professor of Clinical and Health Psychology, University College London
ANDY SHIH, Senior Vice President, Scientific Affairs, Autism Speaks
KARLEE SILVER, President of Targeted Challenges, Grand Challenges Canada
SIMON SOMMER, Head of Research, Jacobs Foundation
TAHA E. TAHA, Professor, Epidemiology and Population, Family and Reproductive Health Sciences, Bloomberg School of Public Health, Johns Hopkins University
SUSAN WALKER, Professor of Nutrition, and Director, Tropical Medicine Research Institute, Epidemiology Research Unit, University of the West Indies
SARA WATSON, National Director, ReadyNation, Council for a Strong America
AMALIA WAXMAN, Consultant
QUENTIN WODON, Advisor, Human Development Network, World Bank
HIROKAZU YOSHIKAWA, Courtney Sale Ross University Professor of Globalization and Education, New York University

Forum Staff

KIMBER BOGARD, Director, Forum on Investing in Young Children Globally
CHARLEE ALEXANDER, Associate Program Officer
CARRIE VERGEL DE DIOS, Senior Program Assistant
FAYE HILLMAN, Financial Officer
PATRICK W. KELLEY, Director, Board on Global Health

Consultant

JOCELYN WIDMER, University of Florida

BOARD ON GLOBAL HEALTH[1]

[1] The National Academies of Sciences, Engineering, and Medicine's boards do not review or approve individual products. The responsibility for the content of the workshop summary rests with the workshop rapporteur and the institution.

BOARD ON CHILDREN, YOUTH, AND FAMILIES[1]

[1] The National Academies of Sciences, Engineering, and Medicine's boards do not review or approve individual products. The responsibility for the content of the workshop summary rests with the workshop rapporteur and the institution.

Reviewers

This workshop summary has been reviewed in draft form by individuals chosen for their diverse perspectives and technical expertise. The purpose of this independent review is to provide candid and critical comments that will assist the institution in making its published workshop summary as sound as possible and to ensure that the workshop summary meets institutional standards for objectivity, evidence, and responsiveness to the study charge. The review comments and draft manuscript remain confidential to protect the integrity of the process. We wish to thank the following individuals for their review of this workshop summary:

Radosveta Dimitrova, Stockholm University, Sweden
Deepa Grover, UNICEF
Venita Kaul, Ambedkar University, Delhi
Mark Miller, Fogarty International Center, National Institutes of Health

Although the reviewers listed above have provided many constructive comments and suggestions, they did not see the final draft of the workshop summary before its release. The review of this workshop summary was overseen by **Floyd Bloom,** Professor Emeritus of The Scripps Research Institute. He was responsible for making certain that an independent examination of this workshop summary was carried out in accordance with institutional procedures and that all review comments were carefully considered. Responsibility for the final content of this workshop summary rests entirely with the rapporteur and the institution.

Acknowledgments

The planning committee and project staff deeply appreciate the many valuable contributions from individuals who assisted us with this project. First, we offer our profound thanks to all of the presenters and discussants at the workshop who gave so generously of their time and expertise. These individuals are listed in full in the workshop agenda in Appendix B. We are also grateful to the many participants who attended the workshop. The engagement of all those in attendance was robust and vital to the success of the event.

In addition, the forum wishes to recognize the sponsors that supported this activity. Financial support for this project was provided by Autism Speaks; the Bernard van Leer Foundation; The Bill & Melinda Gates Foundation; the Doris Duke Charitable Foundation; the Fraser Mustard Institute for Human Development; Fundação Maria Cecilia Souto Vidigal; Grand Challenges Canada; HighScope Educational Research Foundation; the Inter-American Development Bank; the Jacobs Foundation; Lumos; the National Institutes of Health—Fogarty International Center, the National Institute of Child Health and Human Development, and the National Institute of Mental Health; Nestlé Nutrition Institute; Open Society Institute–Budapest Foundation; ReadyNation; the Robert Wood Johnson Foundation; the Society for Research in Child Development; UNICEF; U.S. Agency for International Development; U.S. Centers for Disease Control and Prevention; and the World Bank.

A NOTE ABOUT THE COVER ART

The Forum on Investing in Young Children Globally is committed to confronting the challenges and harnessing the opportunities surrounding the global nature of integrating the science of health, education, nutrition, and social protection. One of the ways the forum has committed itself to being global in scope is through the workshops that occur in different regions throughout the world. The cover design is intended to embrace the diversity in place, culture, challenges, and opportunities associated with forum activities at each of the workshops, but this global trajectory is done keeping in mind the momentum that comes in connecting these diverse locales to one another through the work of the forum. The bright orange dot represents the location of the workshop this report summarizes, and the lighter orange dots represent workshop locations across the first 3 years of the forum. The dotted orange line suggests that the forum will link what was gleaned from the convening activities from this workshop to the next. We would like to thank Jocelyn Widmer for her contributions to the cover design.

Contents

1

Introduction and Overview[1]

The United Nations Sustainable Development Goals (UN SDGs) for 2015–2030 strive for a world that is "just, equitable, and inclusive," in which everyone receives care, education, and opportunities to thrive (UN General Assembly, 2015). Yet many children are living on the margins of society, face multiple disadvantages, and are excluded from full participation in all that life has to offer. To examine the science, economics, and politics of investing in the health, education, nutrition, and social protection of children at the margins, the Forum on Investing in Young Children Globally (iYCG Forum) held a workshop in Prague, Czech Republic, on November 3–4, 2015, titled, "Reaching and Investing in Children at the Margins." Held in partnership with the Open Society Foundations and the International Step by Step Association (ISSA), the workshop convened a diverse group of stakeholders from around the world for 2 days of discussion. Individual workshop participants sought to

1. bring to the foreground a scientific perspective of children at the margins, and

[1] The planning committee's role was limited to planning the workshop. The workshop summary has been prepared by the rapporteur (with the assistance of Kimber Bogard and Carrie Vergel de Dios) as a factual account of what occurred at the workshop. Statements, recommendations, and opinions expressed are those of individual presenters and participants and are not necessarily endorsed or verified by the National Academies of Sciences, Engineering, and Medicine. They should not be construed as reflecting any group consensus.

2. explore how discrimination and social exclusion affect early development, focusing on vulnerable populations such as children living outside of family care; children from diverse ethnic and linguistic backgrounds such as Roma; children with developmental delays and disabilities; and refugee, immigrant, and migrant children.

Box 1-1 provides the full statement of task for the workshop. In providing an overview of the iYCG Forum, Zulfiqar Bhutta stated that the global agenda has shifted from saving lives and ensuring basic rights for individuals to focusing on sustainability, holistic human development, and the numerous factors affecting health and well-being. Ann Masten[2] added three additional global trends: (1) a shift from focusing on survival to healthy development and thriving; (2) a growing body of science surrounding healthy child development and well-being; and (3) a convergence of goals among multiple stakeholders that necessitates coordination and integration at the highest levels. Masten stated that these trends align with the forum's vision of ensuring decision makers around the world use the best available evidence to optimize the well-being of children and their lifelong potential. A full overview of the forum is presented in Box 1-2.

In her opening remarks, Nives Milinovic[3] stated that for the first time, early childhood is on the global agenda. The UN SDG targets for quality standards, equity, gender parity, nutrition, health, and a qualified workforce provide clear guidance for how much countries still need to achieve for children and families since the expiration of the Millennium Development Goals (MDGs), she said. Milinovic highlighted the conflict in Syria, which has resulted in the global movement of more than 4 million people fleeing violence and persecution since 2011—an unprecedented amount—as an example of where more can be done. She remarked that along the "refugee road" in Europe—one of the richest regions in the world—children fleeing persecution in Syria are "hungry, sick, sleeping on the frozen ground, and face an uncertain future." In responding to this crisis, she underscored the need for the global community to bridge research, policy, financing, and practice, emphasizing that while investing in people is sometimes the hardest and longest investment, it is also the most necessary. She closed with the motto of ISSA's Romani Early Years Network, "No more lost generations."

[2] Ann Masten is the Distinguished McKnight University Professor, Institute of Child Development, University of Minnesota.

[3] Nives Milinovic is president of the ISSA board.

BOX 1-1
Workshop Statement of Task

An ad hoc committee will plan and conduct an interactive public workshop featuring presentations and discussions that highlight the science and economics of investing in children at the margins of society by investing in their health, education, nutrition, and social protection. This workshop, the sixth in the Forum on Investing in Young Children Globally series, brings to the foreground a scientific perspective on children at the margins. The workshop will include a critical review of the implementation of the Convention on the Rights of the Child as it applies to young children, as well as an exploration of how discrimination and social exclusion affect early development. Subsequent sessions will focus on new information about children living at the margins. The effect of discrimination on young children from under-resourced groups will be explored using the example of Roma children in Europe.

The results of the workshop will inform research, policy, and practice in the region as well as globally. The committee will identify specific topics to be addressed, develop the agenda, select and invite speakers and other participants, and moderate the discussions. A workshop summary and brief workshop summary of the presentations and discussions at the workshop will be prepared by a designated rapporteur in accordance with institutional guidelines. Communications and dissemination products will be drawn from workshop proceedings.

WORKSHOP OVERVIEW

Sarah Klaus[4] stated that this workshop in Prague provided an opportunity for the iYCG Forum to focus on what the science and experience reveal about investing in children at the margins, with the hope of generating guidance on developing and implementing better policies and services. The workshop was grounded in child rights and explored the effects marginalization has on various groups around the world, including children living outside of family care; children from diverse ethnic and linguistic backgrounds such as Roma; children with developmental delays and disabilities; and refugee, immigrant, and migrant children. Presenters also explored the use of measurement to support early childhood development.

ORGANIZATION OF THE WORKSHOP SUMMARY REPORT

Following this introduction and overview, Chapter 2 provides an introduction to young children's rights and highlights the intersection of the UN Convention on the Rights of the Child (UN CRC) and the UN

[4] Sarah Klaus is director of the Open Society Foundations' Early Childhood Program.

BOX 1-2
The Forum on Investing in Young Children Globally

The Forum on Investing in Young Children Globally (iYCG Forum)—a collaboration between the National Academies of Sciences, Engineering, and Medicine's Board on Global Health and Board on Children, Youth, and Families—was established with the goal to integrate knowledge with action in regions around the world to inform evidence-based, strategic investments in young children. The iYCG Forum is a collaboration of experts working to ensure that investments in the world's children are informed by integrative science and are a top priority on the policy agenda, both globally and nationally. The iYCG Forum is dedicated to ensuring that decision makers around the world use the best science and evidence for investing to optimize the well-being of children and their lifelong potential. The iYCG Forum's main objectives are to explore the importance of an integrated science of healthy child development through age 8; share examples of models of program implementation at scale and financing across social protection, education, health, and nutrition; promote global dialogue on investing in young children; and catalyze opportunities for intersectoral coordination at local, national, and global levels. The iYCG Forum aims to identify and communicate best practices in the translation of science and evidence into programs and policies that improve the lives and potential of young children around the world.

Five previous workshops focused on the cost of inaction; financing investments in young children; scaling up those investments; looking at existing platforms to support investments; and examining how families and communities invest in young children globally. Brief summaries of the workshops are available at the forum's website (http://hmd.nationalacademies.org/activities/children/investingyoungchildrenglobally.aspx), and full summaries are available from the National Academies Press (http://www.nap.edu).

SDGs. Chapter 3 explores how institutionalization and living outside of family care affects early child development. Chapter 4 discusses how discrimination and social exclusion affect young Romani children. Chapter 5 provides practitioner and policy perspectives on including children with developmental delays and disabilities in research and policy agendas around the world. Using the conflict in Syria as a backdrop, Chapter 6 includes presentations of refugee, immigrant, and migrant children. Chapter 7 examines efforts to combine the science of child development with quality measurement to support early childhood programs and policies. The chapter compares four assessment and monitoring tools across health, education, nutrition, and social protection. Appendix A contains a list of abbreviations and acronyms; Appendix B provides the workshop agenda; and Appendix C lists biographical sketches of the workshop speakers.

2

Young Children's Rights and the Effects of Discrimination

Jonathan Todres[1] discussed the importance of the 1989 United Nations Convention on the Rights of the Child (UN CRC), detailed how this global commitment intersects with the United Nations Sustainable Development Goals (UN SDGs), and outlined key considerations in advancing children's rights and well-being. The UN CRC, a treaty to which every country in the world is a party except the United States, has four foundational principles. These principles establish that children have a right to life, survival, and development (Article 6); to have decision makers and policy makers consider their best interests (Article 3); to fully participate in actions and decisions that affect their lives (Article 12); and that children are entitled to the rights enshrined in the UN CRC without discrimination (Article 2). According to Todres, the UN CRC is particularly important because it establishes a legal mandate. In essence, countries must protect and provide for their children not on moral grounds, but because they are legally compelled to do so.

The UN CRC contains a range of substantive provisions that cover health, education, nutrition, and social protection, as well as numerous other issues. As stated by Todres, like other human rights treaties, the UN CRC has reporting requirements that require governments to report to the Committee on the Rights of the Child every 5 years on the steps they are taking to provide for children; what progress is being made; and what

[1] Jonathan Todres is a professor of law at the Georgia State University College of Law in the United States.

obstacles have been encountered. Based on these reports and input from civil society, the committee offers recommendations for action, which in many occasions have spurred legislation that led to improvements for children. For Todres, this reporting procedure provides a built-in monitoring and evaluation function. Although he cautioned against causation, Todres said that in the era of the UN CRC—since 1989—there have been a number of changes in countries' laws—both at the constitutional level and in other national laws—that have significantly advanced child rights and well-being (Adamson et al., 2007). In addition, Todres explained that data show an improvement in outcomes for many children, such as a decrease in under-5 mortality from 12 million per year in 1990 to less than 6 million in 2015 (WHO, 2016) and a reduction in the number of children out of school and involved in child labor. Another benefit of the UN CRC, Todres said, is that it creates a dedicated process for children that elevates the special care and attention needed for this vulnerable population; other human rights systems combine adults and children, sometimes including children as an afterthought. He did note some limitations in the convention, citing enforcement issues and the opportunity for misinterpretation of the "best interests of the child" provision.

THE INTERSECTION OF THE UN CRC AND THE UN SDGs

When comparing the UN SDGs to the UN CRC, Todres found significant overlap and parallel mandates. As an example, Target 1.1 of UN SDG Goal 1: "End poverty in all its forms everywhere," aims to eradicate extreme poverty by 2030. Article 27 of the UN CRC likewise requires governments to recognize that children have the right to an adequate standard of living with a focus on nutrition, clothing, and housing. UN SDG Target 1.4 emphasizes the importance of property ownership and inheritance rights. UN CRC Article 2 has relevant requirements to prohibit discrimination that, when used in the context of children orphaned by AIDS, can help prevent property grabbing and ensure entitlement to property and inheritance rights. Looking at UN SDG 4: "Ensure inclusive and equitable quality education and promote lifelong learning opportunities for all," Todres highlighted several relevant UN CRC articles (as outlined in Table 2-1). Article 28 compels countries to make primary education compulsory and free to all children; make secondary education available and accessible to every child; make higher education accessible to all on the basis of capacity; and take steps to encourage attendance and reduce dropout rates. Article 29 states that education should be directed to the fullest development of the child, with respect for human rights and fundamental freedoms, gender equality, and other targets contained in the UN SDGs. For Todres, there are substantive opportunities to combine

TABLE 2-1 Comparison of SDG 4 to UN CRC Articles 2, 28, 29, and 42

UN SDG Goal	UN SDG Targets	UN CRC Articles
Goal 4—Ensure inclusive and equitable quality education and promote lifelong learning opportunities for all.	Target 4.1—By 2030, ensure that all girls and boys complete free, equitable, and quality primary and secondary education leading to relevant and effective learning outcomes.	Article 28—States parties recognize the right of the child to education, and with . . . equal opportunity.
	Target 4.2—By 2030, ensure that all girls and boys have access to quality early childhood development, care and preprimary education so they are ready for primary education.	Article 2—Nondiscrimination
	Target 4.7—By 2030, ensure that all learners acquire the knowledge and skills needed to promote sustainable development, including, among others, through education for sustainable development and sustainable lifestyles, human rights, gender equality, promotion of a culture of peace and nonviolence, global citizenship and appreciation of cultural diversity and of culture's contribution to sustainable development.	Article 29—Education shall be directed to the development of the child's fullest potential and to respect for human rights, gender equality, etc.
		Article 42—State parties will undertake to make the rights in the CRC widely known.

NOTE: CRC = Convention of the Rights of the Child; SDG = Sustainable Development Goal; UN = United Nations.
SOURCES: UN General Assembly, 2015; UNICEF, 1989.

the UN SDGs and the UN CRC to advance the rights and well-being of children.

KEY CONSIDERATIONS WHEN ADVANCING CHILDREN'S RIGHTS

Todres closed his talk by presenting five key considerations when advancing children's rights and well-being.

The Time-Sensitive Nature of Children's Rights

Todres stated that in some cases, denial of the right to health care for an adult for a relatively short period of time (e.g., 2 years), might not be as great a detriment as it would for a child. For many children, poor health care and nutrition for a brief duration can significantly affect their growth and development. Likewise, being out of school for a short period might prevent a child from ever returning to school, drastically altering their life course. Todres pointed to internally displaced persons and the large number of refugees worldwide, 41 percent of whom are children, who often have lengthy stays in refugee camps. He urged decision makers to be cognizant of the sensitive early development period and to realize that interruptions in access to services might have critical long-term consequences.

Discrimination

According to Todres, well-documented evidence shows the detrimental effects discrimination has on a child's psychological well-being, scholastic achievement, and social-emotional growth. In particular, he focused on multiple forms of discrimination and intersectionality, citing Kimberlé Crenshaw, who coined the term *intersectionality* and asserted that multiple forms of discrimination cannot be considered independently. Instead, one must consider their interactions, which reinforce each other (Crenshaw, 1989). Drawing on research on Romani girls, Todres explained how a young Romani girl may be discriminated against because she is a girl, a Romani, and a child, and that all of these streams of discrimination will disadvantage her by denying or limiting access to institutions, education, health care, and the justice system (Ravnbøl, 2009). For Todres, considering multiple forms of discrimination can help inform thinking about marginalized communities.

The Interrelationship Among Rights

It is well-accepted that rights are interrelated and interdependent and have horizontal and vertical relationships, said Todres, but greater attention must be given to the effect of these interrelationships. An example of a horizontal relationship is the effect poor health has on school attendance and education. Removing school fees is a good start for providing access to education and securing education rights, but many marginalized children still cannot attend school because of other barriers such as poorer health or lack of access to health care, resulting in higher absenteeism from school. Todres called for a more holistic approach to address health, education, and other rights. He used the relationship between women's rights and children's rights as a notable example of a vertical relationship. As women bear the *de facto* primary responsibility for child care in many countries, the ability for a woman to realize her rights, educational opportunities, and employment opportunities has a direct effect on her children.

Mainstreaming

Drawing on the UN SDGs targets for infrastructure development and sustainable development, Todres said that decision makers often discuss children in relation to health and education, but they should realize that decisions made about infrastructure, transportation, and other sectors also affect the lives of children. To ensure child well-being features prominently in a country's agenda, he recommends ensuring that governments account for children's rights at the design, implementation, and monitoring and evaluation stages of law, policy, and programming in all sectors (Todres, 2011). He also added the importance of involving children in these processes.

Maturity

Children are often making mature decisions in the face of adversity, such as Syrian refugee children or unaccompanied minors crossing from Central America to the United States (Todres, 2014). According to Todres, sometimes children's decision-making processes or opinions are not expressed in an adultlike manner, causing adults and decision makers to dismiss them (Todres, 2014). However, being open to children's insights about their lives and experiences can improve programming, Todres said. He again referenced Article 12 of the UN CRC, which gives the child a right to participate in decisions that affect their lives, based on the presumption that any child capable of forming a view should have the opportunity to express that view and have it adequately considered.

3

The Effects of Institutionalization and Living Outside of Family Care on Children's Early Development

Orphans and children living outside of family care are an extremely vulnerable population, often exposed to poverty, stigma, physical and sexual violence, and a lack of educational resources, according to research cited by Vesna Kutlesic (Cluver et al., 2013; Morantz et al., 2013).[1] Other research indicates it is important to explore whether these children were first exposed to traumatic life events while living with their families, or subsequent to separation from their families to an out-of-family placement (e.g., an institution or foster care), or after ending up homeless and living on the street (Atwoli et al., 2014; Gray et al., 2015; Li et al., 2009; Whetten et al., 2014). Regardless of the timing of traumatic life events, Kutlesic emphasized the importance of building on the strengths of these children, eliminating stigma, and fostering their growth and well-being through their participation in evidence-based, multidisciplinary interventions aimed at improving their health, education, and psychosocial development.

Low- and middle-income countries (LMICs) are home to an estimated 132 million single and double orphans (cases in which either one or both parents are deceased), 95 percent of whom are over the age of 5 (UNICEF, 2015). Further research estimates that more than 8 million children around the world grow up in institutions (Csaky, 2009). Additionally, UNICEF estimates that there are tens of millions of street children who need care,

[1] Vesna Kutlesic is director of the Office of Global Health at the *Eunice Kennedy Shriver* National Institute for Child Health and Human Development.

and that this number is increasing (UNICEF, 2009). Caring for these vulnerable children therefore presents a complex problem that requires evidence-based solutions, a continuum of care, and placements for children with a diverse set of health, education, and psychosocial needs, said Kutlesic. Each model of care (institutionalization, family-based care, etc.) has its strengths and weaknesses, with primary goals being to provide a quality environment for children, opportunities for learning and growth, and protection from harm.

According to Kutlesic, when families are stressed and unable to care for a child or are at risk of harming a child, it is important to consider the child's age, health, and developmental needs when determining an optimal living arrangement and support services. For children under age 2, research conducted by the Bucharest Early Intervention Project, the St. Petersburg–USA Orphanage Research Team, and others has focused on large hospital-style institutions employing shift workers with minimal interactions with residing infants and children, with results demonstrating powerful negative effects on the infant brain and other aspects of child development (Nelson et al., 2014; St. Petersburg–USA Orphanage Research Team, 2008). When these infants were later placed with trained, paid, and supervised foster parents, some brain and other developmental improvements have been observed, while others appear irreversible (Fox et al., 2011; St. Petersburg–USA Orphanage Research Team, 2008).

However, other studies of long-term outcomes of children placed in institutional care have found more nuanced positive outcomes, particularly among children over age 5 and those living in low-income countries (Embleton et al., 2014; Merz et al., 2013; Whetten et al., 2014). For example, the Positive Outcomes for Orphans study conducted in Cambodia, Ethiopia, India, Kenya, and Tanzania has found that children living in institutional settings scored as well or better than their counterparts in family-based care across measures such as physical and emotional well-being. According to Kutlesic, these data do not suggest that institutions are preferential to family settings. Rather the data suggest that children living in communities that are in the process of developing well-trained family and foster care placements have demonstrated positive psychosocial adjustment and developmental gains when placed in smaller institutions (such as group homes) that are well-organized and contain a strong educational component. She also cautioned that as part of reform projects aimed at the deinstitutionalization of children to family, foster care, and adoptive placements, it is important to have parallel efforts aimed at caregiver training, community health and social services, and strengthening the foster care system. These efforts reduce the risk of failed child placements and the unintended consequence of contributing to the growing numbers of street children, she said.

Kutlesic closed by suggesting that in order for children who are not able to live with their families to be provided with the opportunity for optimal developmental outcomes, it is important to provide high-quality living environments that are tailored to the needs of individual children and include opportunities for learning and growth, well-trained caregivers, and appropriate adult-to-child ratios, regardless of placement setting.

THE EFFECTS OF INSTITUTIONALIZATION ON BEHAVIORAL DEVELOPMENT

In 2003, the European Commission Daphne Program funded a survey to examine the risk of harm to children under the age of 3 years living in institutions across 54 European countries (Browne et al., 2006). Kevin Browne and his team focused on behavioral consequences of institutionalization compared to family-based care, primarily in western and central European countries of the European Union (EU).[2] At the beginning of the study, survey results showed that some countries had no children in institutional care,[3] compared to the Czech Republic which institutionalized six children per 1,000, the highest figure in Europe. At the time, 44,000 children under 3 years old were in institutions across Europe and Central Asia; 23,000 children under 3 were in institutions in the EU member states and could spend up to 18 hours per day in their cribs. Browne's findings showed that institutions negatively affect a child's social behavior and interaction with others, as well as negatively affecting the formation of emotional attachments. Additionally, being institutionalized was linked to poor cognitive performance and language deficits. To combat the detrimental effects of institutionalization on young children, UNICEF launched a deinstitutionalization campaign after the United Nations (UN) General Assembly released guidelines saying that no child under 3 years of age should be in institutional care.

In 2013, Browne said that while some countries significantly reduced the number of children under 3 in institutions during the previous decade, others increased their number, as evidenced by 46 out of 54 country responses to the survey. Increases were seen in Austria,[4] Albania, Malta, Moldova, Croatia, Bosnia and Herzegovina, Poland, and Tajikistan (arranged in order of largest percent increase) despite significant investment from nongovernmental organizations (NGOs) (Browne and Chou,

[2] Kevin Browne is director of the Center for Forensic and Family Psychology at the University of Nottingham, United Kingdom.

[3] Countries with no children in institutional care included Slovenia and the United Kingdom.

[4] Browne hypothesized that the additional three children in Austrian institutions are refugee children from abroad rather than Austrian nationals.

2015). Countries that significantly reduced the number of children in residential care were Belgium, Czech Republic, Slovakia, Spain, Romania, Finland, Belarus, Estonia, Russia, The Netherlands, and Bulgaria (arranged in order of largest percent decrease) (Browne and Chou, 2015). Browne highlighted an increase in foster care, stating that the majority of children are now in family-based care because countries have made efforts to reduce the numbers in institutional care. He noted that more work has to be done, however, and that several countries still lag behind in developing a legitimate family-based care system, notably Belgium, Italy, and Spain. Although the Czech Republic currently has high numbers of children in institutions compared to other countries in Europe, Browne commended the country's efforts to reduce institutionalization by 22 children per 10,000 (Browne and Chou, 2015).

Reasons for institutionalization varied and have changed little since 2003, according to Browne's research. In Western European countries, 4 percent of children were institutionalized because they were abandoned, another 4 percent were disabled, and 68 percent were abused and neglected. In Eastern Europe and Central Asia, children were more likely to be institutionalized because of disability (23 percent), abandonment (33 percent), and because they were abused or neglected (14 percent), according to Browne (2009). He noted that abandoned children, children with disabilities, and those from ethnic groups face more discrimination than children institutionalized for other reasons. In the Czech Republic and Slovakia, a significant proportion of children in institutions are of Romani origins and a significant number have disabilities. Browne also proposed that several societal influences have led to the development of institutional care, including

- A lack of community nurses and social workers, who, according to research, are the best actors to prevent abandonment and violence in the community (Browne, 2009; Hamilton-Giachritsis and Browne, 2012)
- A lack of home-based assessments of children in need and their families
- A lack of free universal prevention services to reduce child abuse, neglect, and abandonment
- Weak targeted interventions with families at high risk of child abuse, neglect, and abandonment
- Slow development of high-quality foster care systems

In closing, Browne suggested the provision of high-quality foster care, community services for families in need, and daycare facilities for children with and without disabilities to reduce the number of children in institutions. He recommended residential care only for children who may harm themselves or others, as well as an increased number of mother–baby units in institutions when community services do not exist.

THE BUCHAREST EARLY INTERVENTION PROJECT

According to Anne Berens,[5] social policies under Nicolae Ceauşescu's authoritarian rule of Romania from 1965 to 1989—such as a ban on contraception and a tax on families without children—coupled with widespread poverty led to rising fertility and high rates of child abandonment into state institutions. At the end of this regime in 1989, there were an estimated 170,000 children in institutions. It is in this historical context that researchers developed the Bucharest Early Intervention Project, a longitudinal study in Romania that began in 2000 with ongoing follow-up today. The project has three aims:

1. Examine the effects of institutionalization on the brain and behavioral development of young children.
2. Determine if observed negative effects can be remediated by placing children in high-quality foster care.
3. Improve the welfare of Romanian children by establishing foster care as an alternative to institutionalization.

Berens reported that in 2000 many political leaders questioned whether institutions were actually harmful for young children. Although baseline findings showed that children in institutions had significantly lower cognitive development scores than children who were not in institutions (Smyke et al., 2007), some believed that deficits among institutionalized children existed prior to institutionalization rather than developing due to residential care. For example, children placed in institutions may have been exposed to risk factors that led to placement in residential care such as exposure to fetal drugs and alcohol, or mothers who could not access prenatal care.

In response to these questions, Bucharest Early Intervention Project researchers designed a randomized control trial to control for environmental and background differences between children and examine the treatment effects incurred from high-quality foster care. When the project started, there was no national foster care system, only local initiatives largely supported by NGOs, said Berens. Therefore, researchers recruited and trained 58 foster families, the maximum amount possible based on funding from their grant.

[5] Anne Berens is the Julius B. Richmond Fellow at Harvard University in the United States.

Researchers randomly assigned 136 children from state-run institutions into two groups (keeping siblings together): children who would move from an institution to foster families (foster care group) and those who would remain in institutions (institutional group). Sixty-eight children were assigned to the foster care group and 68 to the institutional group; 72 children from the community who had never been institutionalized comprised the control sample and were referred to as the "never institutionalized group." According to Berens, the mean age of the sample prior to the intervention was 21.6 months and the mean age at placement into foster care was 22 months. Researchers conducted follow-up assessments at 30, 42, and 54 months, and 8 and 12 years. Age 16 follow-up was being conducted at the time of the meeting.

Bucharest Early Intervention Project researchers examined a wide range of outcomes: cognition, neurodevelopment (electroencephalogram [EEG], magnetic resonance imaging, and event-related potentials), psychopathology, physical development, social skills, attachment, language, temperament, autonomic and hypothalamic–pituitary–adrenal function, and genetics and epigenetics.[6] In analyses of cognition, researchers found that the foster care group had significant improvements in intelligence quotient (IQ) at ages 30, 42, and 54 months compared to the institutionalized group (Fox et al., 2011). Taking into account the age at which a child was placed in foster care, data showed evidence of greater gains for IQ in younger children, particularly those placed before 24 months old (Nelson et al., 2007). Examining EEG patterns, researchers found that children placed into foster care after 24 months of age had brain activity indistinguishable from the institutionalized group, whereas children placed before 24 months had EEG patterns that were indistinguishable from the never institutionalized group (Vanderwert et al., 2010). The study also found high rates of psychiatric disorders—around 38 percent—in the institutionalized group and increased rates of behavioral difficulties such as attention deficit hyperactivity disorder, externalizing symptoms, and aggression (Humphreys et al., 2015).

Finally, Berens stated that timing effects were seen across a number of domains with evidence of greater recovery of the foster care group if placed before 12, 15, 20, and 24 months. In addition to IQ and brain function, differences were noted in language, social skills, inhibitory control, and attachment (Almas et al., 2012; Bos et al., 2010, 2011; McDermott et al., 2013; Vanderwert et al., 2010; Windsor et al., 2011) (see Figure 3-1). Importantly, Berens noted that positive effects in the foster care group

[6] Berens focused her presentation on cognition, neurodevelopment, and psychopathology, and encouraged participants to visit the project website for a discussion of findings on the other measures: http://www.bucharestearlyinterventionproject.org.

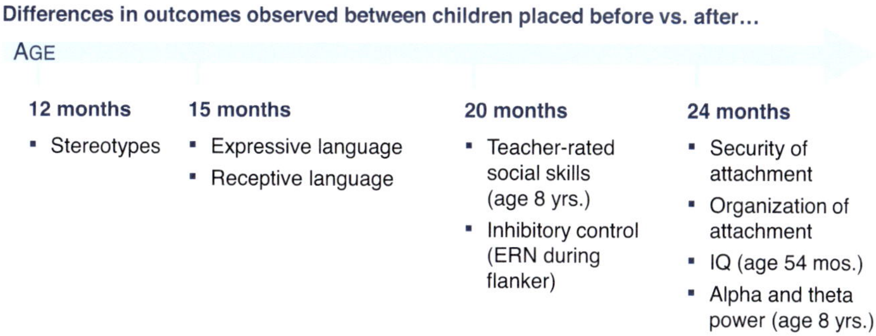

FIGURE 3-1 Effect modification by age at foster care placement suggests multiple sensitive periods across developmental domains.
NOTE: ERN = error-related negativity; IQ = intelligence quotient.
SOURCES: Almas et al., 2012; Bos et al., 2010, 2011; McDermott et al., 2013; Nelson et al., 2007; Vanderwert et al., 2010; Windsor et al., 2011.

were true only for children who had stable placements; children who had disrupted foster care often fared worse than the institutionalized group.

LUMOS FOUNDATION'S MODEL OF DEINSTITUTIONALIZATION IN MOLDOVA

Irina Malanciuc presented Lumos Foundation's successful deinstitutionalization model in Moldova. Formerly part of the Soviet Union, Moldova is a young country—24 years old—with a population of over 3.5 million people, a fifth of whom are children (up to age 18).[7,8] According to Malanciuc, the country is very poor with an underdeveloped economy.[9] Due to high rates of poverty, parents often leave children in care of relatives and neighbors and go in search of work in other countries. Based on the study carried out by Lumos in its pilot regions in Moldova, it was estimated that 20 percent of children live without their parents (Lumos, 2009). There are many children with disabilities who live in institutions and who are victims of neglect and abuse.

[7] Irina Malanciuc is country director for the Lumos Foundation, Moldova.

[8] Figures provided by the National Bureau of Statistics of the Republic of Moldova. See http://www.statistica.md/newsview.php?l=en&idc=168&id=4779 (accessed February 10, 2016) for more information.

[9] The data from the World Bank indicate that the gross domestic product per capita in Moldova slightly exceeded USD 2,200 in 2014. See http://data.worldbank.org/indicator/NY.GDP.PCAP.CD/countries/MD?display=graph (accessed February 10, 2016) for more information.

Based on a study conducted by the Moldovan government with support from UNICEF, in 2007 Moldova had more than 11,000 children living in 67 residential institutions (Evans, 2013). Of these children, more than 60 percent were older than 12 years old (Evans, 2013). According to Malanciuc, this fact helped the authorities understand that through prevention of institutionalization, support of children who leave residential care because they exceed the age limit, and reintegration of children into families, it was possible to change the system. With an aim to reduce the number of children in institutions by 50 percent by 2012, as targeted in the National Strategy and Action Plan on the residential child care system reform for 2007–2012, Lumos Moldova joined the efforts of authorities and NGOs to decrease the number of children placed in residential care and implemented Lumos' 10-step model for deinstitutionalization, as presented in Box 3-1.

By implementing the National Strategy and Action Plan, the number of children in institutions in Moldova decreased by 62 percent by 2012. Through the development of social services, the creation of alternatives to institutional care, family support, community-based services, and intersectorial coordination at the central and local levels, Lumos Moldova, in partnership with UNICEF, Hope and Homes for Children, and Every Child, reduced the number of children in institutions to fewer than 3,000 by the end of 2014. A large part of this decrease was due to the development of inclusive education, said Malanciuc. In 2010, only 8 percent of children with disabilities were enrolled in mainstream education; in 2014, this number climbed to 50 percent.[10] Also, most children returned to their families, who were involved in the deinstitutionalization process from the beginning.

Lumos supported the development of a normative framework for child protection and the creation of new social and educational services. The foundation assisted authorities in closing six residential institutions from its pilot regions, reintegrating children into their families, and supporting graduates. Despite reducing the number of children in institutions in Moldova, Malanciuc did note some challenges, namely that Moldova still has children under age 3 living in institutions and that as of 2014, more than half of remaining children in institutions have disabilities and special education needs. Additionally, she highlighted a lack of services for those who leave care. Through creating care opportunities for these children and increasing the number of staff in areas such as social protection and education, Malanciuc is hopeful that the deinstitutionalization process will continue.

[10] Data is estimated based on figures provided by the National Bureau of Statistics of the Republic of Moldova. See http://www.statistica.md/public/files/publicatii_electronice/Educatia/Educatia_RM_2015.pdf (accessed February 10, 2016) for more information.

BOX 3-1
Lumos Foundation's 10-Step Model for Deinstitutionalization

1. Raising awareness—Citing well-documented research, Lumos spreads evidence about the negative effects of institutionalization on children, highlights better alternatives to residential care, describes the process of change, and educates stakeholders about the roles of each actor involved in the deinstitutionalization process.
2. Managing the process—Malanciuc emphasized the importance of this step, as residential institutions are generally housed under different ministries and varying local public authorities. Establishing intersectorial steering committees at the regional level that manage the deinstitutionalization process and providing oversight to these committees is a key strategy for Lumos.
3. Country analysis to assess the current situation and needs.
4. County and residential institution analysis.
5. Service design to support the creation of new, alternative services based on country, county, and institutional analyses.
6. Plan the transfer of resources to support the creation of new services. Malanciuc stated that funding and human resources in very poor countries are directed to residential institutions. Lumos aims to transfer these resources to alternative family and community services to help prevent institutionalization.
7. Preparing and moving children—For Malanciuc, children are the most critical component of the deinstitutionalization process, and it is important to inform them about what is happening, prepare them for change, and allow them to participate in decision making.
8. Preparing and moving personnel—Transferring human resources, goods, and financial services from institutions to alternative services is very difficult, said Malanciuc.
9. Logistical planning for the entire process.
10. Monitoring and evaluation—This step is an important component of deinstitutionalization, said Malanciuc, as the entire process needs to be supervised to determine if the strategic plan needs to be revised based on implementation roadblocks.

SOURCE: Malanciuc, 2015.

TRANSFORMING CHILD CARE SYSTEMS: A CZECH POLICY PERSPECTIVE

Katerina Slesingerova suggested three reasons why transforming the child care system can be a difficult task.[11] First, while most people agree that children need protection, they do not agree on how this should be

[11] Katerina Slesingerova is head of the Department for the Protection of Children's Rights at the Ministry of Labor and Social Affairs in the Czech Republic.

provided. Many times, scientific evidence supporting a path forward is filtered through personal values and beliefs. Second, Slesingerova said children cannot vote for policies that directly affect their lives. Finally, in the Czech Republic, more than half of public funding goes to institutional care; less than 9 percent goes to prevention, and about 40 percent goes to the foster care system.

As in Moldova, Slesingerova said that the child care system is divided among three ministries: the Ministry of Education, which is responsible for children's homes; the Ministry of Health, which manages baby homes; and the Ministry of Labor and Social Affairs, which is responsible for child protection, social work, foster care, and a social security system. This split means that if savings are incurred in institutional care, the money is not reallocated to preventive care or services for families because responsibility for provision of those services lies with another ministry. Slesingerova noted that some changes are occurring to address this limitation such as discussions between the Ministry of Education and the Ministry of Social Affairs to unify administration of the institutions under one ministry. She emphasized that child care systems do not operate in isolation; they interact with other systems, which requires coordination from the lowest to the highest levels in the country. She added that no child care system is perfect, but that change can continue to be made according to new evidence.

BREAKOUT SESSION ON CHILDREN LIVING OUTSIDE OF FAMILY CARE

In addition to the panel presentations, the workshop featured a session in which workshop participants separated into four groups to discuss best practices for reaching children living at the margins of society. According to Browne, who reported out for the breakout session on children living outside of family care, Malanciuc presented a video by the Lumos Foundation titled, "Children Need Families, Not Orphanages" (narrated by the founder, J. K. Rowling), which highlights the science of developmental and psychological effects institutionalized care has on young children, reasons for institutionalization, and how institutionalized care can be prevented by diverting resources to community services. Malanciuc also highlighted "gatekeeping" practices in Moldova in which a committee gathers to discuss potential outcomes of a child's placement into foster care, kinship care, or institutional care. Only after the committee agrees that the placement is in the child's best interest is the child moved. Malanciuc also discussed the practice of placing social workers in maternity units with a high number of births per year in Moldova to reduce abandonment. With this practice, abandonment of children in maternity units dropped by 41 percent, she said (UNICEF, 2005).

Sevdzhihan Eyubova of the Karin Dom Foundation in Bulgaria highlighted a program the foundation implements in partnership with the Tulip Foundation and the Oak Foundation to prevent the institutionalization of children with disabilities.[12] Specifically, she said the program is aimed at enhancing the capacity for parents to raise their children with disabilities at home, as well as the capacity of organizations in Bulgaria to encourage a family-centered approach to caring for these children. According to Eyubova, there are two sources of encouragement for parents to institutionalize their children: relatives and medical staff. To curb guidance from medical staff to parents to abandon children, Karin Dom placed psychologists in Bulgarian hospitals to support doctors and nurses. Psychologists offered support to staff delivering children with disabilities and talked through alternatives to institutional care.

Workshop participants also discussed foster care. Topics covered included how to promote good foster care through training, support, and diversification, and the various types of foster care such as short-term foster care, long-term foster care, and emergency foster care. Although breakout group participants attempted to determine if institutional care or foster care is preferable, some participants determined they could not make a fair comparison as they would be comparing apples to oranges.

[12] See https://karindom.org.

4

The Effect of Discrimination and Social Exclusion on Young Romani Children

Estimated at 10–12 million, Roma is Europe's largest ethnic minority group.[1] According to Sarah Klaus, Roma children are a vulnerable population, and their communities are marginalized in many ways. For instance, Klaus reported that there are high levels of infant mortality in Roma communities and the life expectancy for Roma is 8–12 years shorter than the general population in Europe (Rodríguez and Rodríguez, 2009). In addition, as many as 20 percent of the Roma in countries such as Bulgaria never enroll in school (UNICEF, 2011), and only one-third of employment-age Roma are employed (UNDP, 2012). More than 50 percent of Roma in Bulgaria reported experiencing discrimination in the past year (UNDP, 2012).

Klaus stated that although Roma make up a fraction of the population in many countries, Romani children are often overrepresented in institutional care. In Slovakia for example, although Roma account for 9 percent of the total population, 82.5 percent of children in institutional care are of Romani origins (European Roma Rights Center et al., 2011). In Hungary, Roma make up 7 percent of the population, yet 65.9 percent of the population of institutionalized children are of Romani origins (European Roma Rights Center et al., 2011) (see Figure 4-1).

On average, Romani children participate in preschool at half the rate of other children in Europe (Brüggemann, 2012) (see Figure 4-2). According to Klaus, this means that one of the most disadvantaged groups in Europe

[1] See http://www.coe.int/en/web/portal/roma (accessed March 1, 2016).

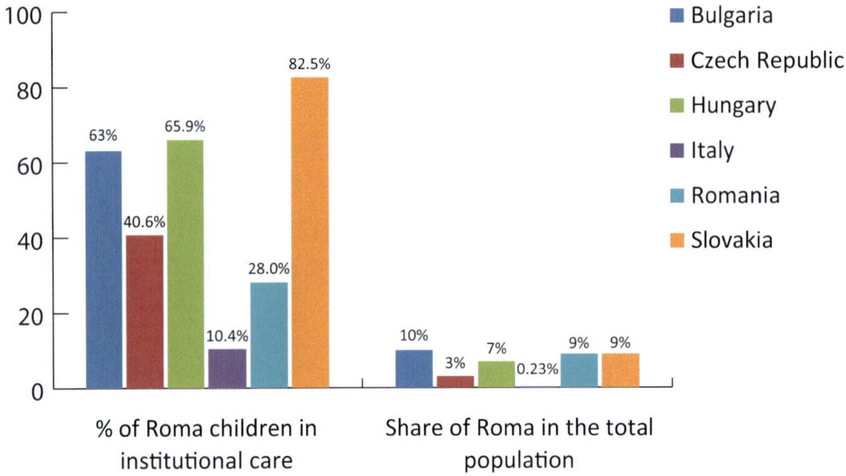

FIGURE 4-1 Roma children in institutional care.
SOURCE: European Roma Rights Centre, Life Sentence: Romani Children in Institutional Care, 2011, p. 7, accessible online at: http://www.errc.org/cms/upload/file/life-sentence-20-june-2011.pdf (accessed March 1, 2016).

has the least access to preschool education. She ventured an assumption that of those Romani children attending preschool, the majority are likely from higher income brackets. Klaus also highlighted the lack of Romani preschool and primary school teachers compared to the Roma population (Klaus, 2014). Household surveys conducted by the World Bank, United Nations Development Programme (UNDP), and the European Commission found that Roma parents would be more comfortable sending their children to school if a Roma teacher was present. In addition to this social barrier, these surveys reveal that the biggest structural barriers to enrolling Romani children in early education programs are the lack of preschools, the distance of preschools from Roma communities, the lack of transportation, and the direct or indirect costs associated with schooling (De Laat et al., 2012).

RISK AND PROTECTIVE FACTORS AFFECTING THE EARLY DEVELOPMENT OF ROMANI CHILDREN

Margareta Matache presented several risk factors and sources of toxic stress that can negatively affect the early development of Romani

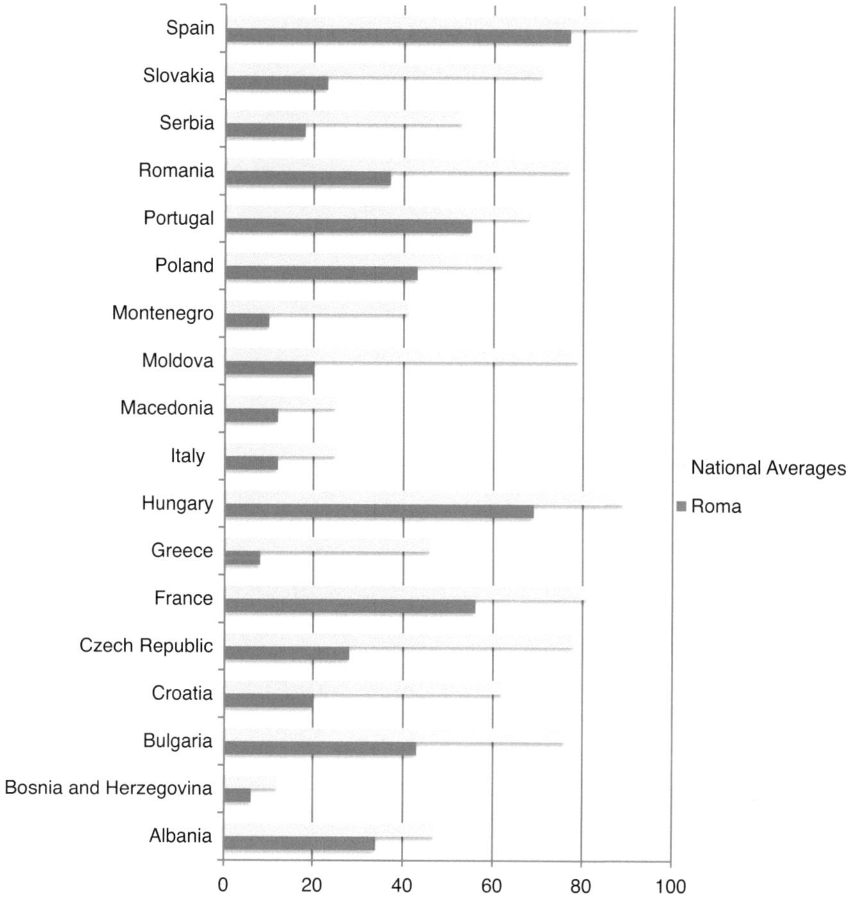

FIGURE 4-2 Preschool attendance rates (percentage) of children aged 3 to entry to formal schooling (age 5 or 6).
SOURCES: UNDP-World Bank Roma survey 2011, UNICEF database 2012 for school year 2010/2011, European Union Agency for Fundamental Rights survey 2011.

children,[2] and she underlined the continuous interactions between sources of vulnerability and resistance to stress and resilience (IOM and NRC, 2000). She argued that understanding when and what type of influence caregivers, schools, and neighborhoods have on a child's development

[2] Margareta Matache is a Roma rights activist from Romania. In 2012 she was awarded a Hauser postdoctoral fellowship at Harvard University, where she currently works as an instructor.

can inform better public policies, teacher training curriculum, and community programs to prevent risks and create better opportunities for all children. Additionally, she indicated that the social and economic context in which children grow up is a strong determinant of inequality.

Romani communities lack resources and experience high rates of discrimination, stigma, and violence (Matache, 2014). Oftentimes, Romani families are geographically separated from the rest of the population, sometimes by walls built by local municipalities, said Matache. This physical separation isolates Roma communities, cutting them off from necessary resources. According to her, 15 percent of Roma families in Romania do not have access to electricity, 36 percent have difficulties obtaining clean drinking water (Fleck, 2008), and more than 40 percent of Romani children suffer from severe malnutrition (Fleck, 2008). Geographic segregation has also affected Romani children's access to education, said Matache. Because of discrimination and stigma faced by Roma, children must attend separate educational facilities. There are very few centers where Romani children can be educated, and at those locations there is low-quality instruction from unqualified teachers, she said. In addition, these institutions generally lack resources and experience very high rates of teacher absenteeism. Moreover, Matache reports that there is discrimination and bullying against Romani children in these schools and centers, as well as a lack of culturally sensitive curricula (Matache, 2014). Romani children enter these environments fearful of how they will be treated by non-Romani teachers and classmates, which influences their attitudes about the institution of education (Matache, 2014). Negative relationships with these groups can lead to psychological difficulties or dropouts, said Matache.

Romani children are also at risk of toxic stress and trauma when exposed to forced evictions, sustained discrimination, and ethnic-based violence, said Matache. In her opinion, this is an understudied, under discussed set of factors that needs more attention from scholars, policy makers, activists, and local authorities. She cited incidences in which non-Romani community members have destroyed Romani houses, killed their animals, and chased away their families, forcing Romani families to sleep in the woods for almost 1 month.[3] Violence against Roma and forced evictions are all too common, said Matache, and leave children with high levels of stress and trauma that affect their emotional, cognitive, and social development.

Matache emphasized that many Romani children are resilient even in very adverse circumstances. However, resilience in the face of discrimination and violence is extremely difficult, she said. The defense mechanisms

[3] See www.romanicriss.org (accessed February 15, 2016).

used by Romani children range from social isolation to forming groups with children from their own ethnic group. According to a focus group of teachers in Romania, "In general, they [Romani children] play with each other" (Focus group, teachers, 2010, Craiova, Romania). Yet there are a few protective factors that mediate the risk factors Romani children are exposed to such as quality maternal care and emotional support from family, peers, and the community (Harwood et al., 2008). Resilience to discrimination is often boosted by psychological optimism, self-esteem, high socioeconomic status, identification with one's in-group, and positive evaluations of the in-group (Son Hing, 2012).

THE ROMA EARLY CHILDHOOD INCLUSION STUDY: RESULTS FROM THE CZECH REPUBLIC

David Greger presented findings from the Roma Early Childhood Inclusion (RECI) report from the Czech Republic.[4] The study was sponsored by the Open Society Foundations, the Roma Education Fund, and UNICEF. According to Greger, researchers found a widespread lack of public child care for children under the age of 3. The Czech Republic has one of the lowest participation rates in child care for children under 3 in the European Union, at less than 3 percent, the second lowest after Poland (Ivatts et al., 2015). Greger and his team also found that there is insufficient kindergarten capacity. Analyses estimate that 27,000 children who apply for kindergarten do not receive a place (Ivatts et al., 2015). Further, there are discriminatory admission criteria that disadvantage Romani families, such as a requirement that mothers of children must be employed in order for children to attend school.

The RECI report highlights inequalities in early childhood education and care in the Czech Republic for disadvantaged Romani children. For instance, children from disadvantaged backgrounds had low levels of participation in preprimary education and delayed enrollment in primary school. Compared to neighboring countries such as Slovakia, Germany, and Austria, which have postponement rates of 8, 8, and 4 percent, respectively, the Czech Republic had a rate of 15 percent for the school year 2013–2014. The evidence also showed that up to 40 percent of Roma children (and other disadvantaged groups) are segregated in special schools, called "practical basic schools," with reduced curricula. According to the Ad Hoc Committee of Experts on Roma Issues, Roma children were 27 times more likely to be placed in a special school than a non-Roma child (Ivatts et al., 2015). Most telling, only 30 percent of Romani boys

---

[4] David Greger is director of the Institute for Research and Development of Education at Charles University in the Czech Republic.

and 50 percent of Romani girls initially enrolled in mainstream schools finished their studies in the same schools; most were instead transferred to a practical basic school (Ivatts et al., 2015).

Chapter 2 of the RECI report discusses findings of Roma children in preschool and kindergarten education. According to Greger, the Czech Republic has 600 excluded localities[5] and there are highly variable rates of preschool enrollment within them, ranging from 10 percent to 100 percent. Overall, the study found that 28 percent of Roma children ages 3 to 6 were enrolled in preschool compared to 64 percent of non-Roma children of the same age (UNDP, 2012). Of those Roma children attending preschool, 14 percent attended schools in which they formed the majority of students; 28 percent attended schools with an even split of Romani and non-Romani children; and more than half attended schools with only a few Romani children. Researchers also found that financial costs associated with kindergarten presented a significant barrier for Romani parents to enroll their children in school. School fees to attend kindergarten range from CZK300 to CZK600 per month, and meals cost between CZK500 and CZK600 per month. Forty-eight percent of parents said they would definitely send their children to kindergarten if it were free of charge, and another 25 percent would consider the possibility. Twenty-four percent of parents would send their children to kindergarten if meals were covered, and another 24 percent said they would reconsider enrollment if free meals were provided, Greger reported (Ivatts et al., 2015).

A POLICY PERSPECTIVE ON THE EFFECTS OF DISCRIMINATION ON YOUNG ROMANI CHILDREN

Arthur Ivatts highlighted what he felt were important differences in the national contexts of Romania and the Czech Republic.[6] In Romania, he stated that there is free compulsory preprimary education for children ages 5 to 6 for all children, including Roma. Additionally, the National Council for Combating Discrimination is conducting mass trainings for primary school teachers, kindergarten teachers, and school inspectors in antidiscrimination and inclusive practices. In the Czech Republic, Ivatts said there is an ongoing national debate surrounding the introduction of 1 year of free compulsory preschool, alongside legislative initiatives that will facilitate the development of inclusive education.

Focusing on similarities between the countries, Ivatts highlighted similar structural barriers to Romani children's access to quality, unsegre-

[5] Locations with a concentration of persons living in inadequate conditions and inhabiting a physically or symbolically delimited space (Gabal Analysis and Consulting, 2015).

[6] Arthur Ivatts is a senior consultant with the Open Society Foundations.

gated early childhood education in Romania and the Czech Republic. He cited extreme poverty, low family educational capital, social exclusion and geographic marginalization, and dangerous living conditions. Moreover, he stated that Romani families live under conditions of high stress, with neglected infrastructure, and institutionalized racism and discrimination. There is a large body of research that informs how to remove some of these barriers; this research is supported by the UNDP, the World Bank, UNICEF, the Open Society Foundations, and the Roma Education Fund. However, Ivatts remarked that policy makers are largely silent on these issues, making them a "hidden disgrace" of Europe. He believes that the treatment of Roma in Europe comes dangerously close to the criteria for crimes against humanity.

Ivatts recommended policy change in the form of ratified antidiscrimination laws with enforcement mechanisms in place. He recommended new laws on inclusive education with trainings for teachers and adults who work in schools and structured outreach programs for marginalized populations. Furthermore, Ivatts called for programs to reduce poverty and provide free transportation, meals, books, and clothes to children. Finally, he suggested severe penalties for hate speech and discrimination.

A RESEARCH REACTION ON THE EFFECTS OF DISCRIMINATION ON YOUNG ROMANI CHILDREN

Radosveta Dimitrova is a developmental and cross-cultural psychologist conducting research with Roma children and families in Bulgaria and post communist countries and territories, including Albania, the Czech Republic, the Former Yugoslav Republic of Macedonia, Kosovo, Romania, and Serbia.[7] In her research reaction, she focused on two items: what is known about Romani children, and what can be done to support their development and well-being. Dimitrova said that most research focuses on the deficits in the Roma community, such as the challenges and barriers they face and the risk factors that negatively affect child development and later success in life. She instead encouraged researchers and policy makers to focus on the assets in Roma communities and to highlight the protective factors such as strong peer networks and school and community connectedness that promote healthy development. She highlighted that Roma families have the potential for success and that policy makers should build on the strengths already present in Roma communities. She also called for the promotion of culturally informed research, policy, and

[7] Radosveta Dimitrova is the COFAS Forte (the Swedish Research Council for Health, Welfare and Working Life) Marie Curie Fellow and docent at Stockholm University in Sweden.

practice and to engage parents, teachers, and communities at all levels. When asked about Roma leadership, Dimitrova shared an example of a Roma-led organization, Amalipe,[8] that provides educational and training programs in Bulgaria for children and their families.

BREAKOUT SESSION ON THE EFFECTS OF DISCRIMINATION AND SOCIAL EXCLUSION ON YOUNG ROMANI CHILDREN

Stanislav Daniel summarized the discussion of the breakout session on the effects of discrimination and social exclusion on young Romani children.[9] According to him, Bozidar Nikolic of Romanipen in Serbia and Miroslav Sklenka from Step by Step Slovakia discussed grassroots initiatives to support Romani children by working with local professionals, paraprofessionals, parents, and children. They stated that their nongovernmental organizations (NGOs) invest in local capacity as a way to ensure sustainability; once the NGOs lay the groundwork, they expect the government to take over the efforts and scale up programs. One breakout participant highlighted an initiative in Ukraine where, for the first time, Roma NGOs met with state and regional administrators to discuss community needs. Another participant noted, however, that even when municipalities sign memorandums of cooperation with Roma communities, they sometimes do not fulfill their obligations to provide for these communities.

Some breakout group participants considered the increasing number of Roma NGOs and Roma activism as a type of Roma movement, a movement that was not present less than a decade ago. They encouraged workshop participants to consider the activities of these numerous organizations as a greater whole, rather than viewing them individually. During this discussion, participants also mentioned the importance of active involvement, stating that it is important for the local community to feel that programs and services are successful and add value to their situation. If communities are invested in the efforts, some participants thought that this would lead to sustainability. To continue providing for Roma children and families, a few breakout participants urged improvements in quality of service and intersectorial coordination.

---

[8] See http://amalipe.com/index.php?nav=About&lang=2 (accessed February 10, 2016).

[9] Stanislav Daniel is program manager and coordinator of ISSA's Romani Early Years Network, based in the Netherlands.

5

Global Efforts to Include Children with Developmental Delays and Disabilities in Research and Policy Agendas

Andy Shih gave a presentation on the South European Autism Network (SEAN).[1] The network, modeled after the World Health Organization's (WHO's) South European Network, involves nine countries in the region: Albania, Bosnia and Herzegovina, Bulgaria, Croatia, Kosovo, Macedonia, Montenegro, Romania, and Slovenia (Turkey is affiliated with the network as an observer country). Every year, national coordinators from each country—who are appointed by each country's minister of health—gather to discuss barriers, successes, and experiences in enhancing the lives of individuals with autism.

From September 2014 to October 2015, the network conducted a Caregiver Needs Study in Albania, Croatia, Macedonia, Romania, and Turkey to understand the parental experience in navigating the system to obtain support for their children. Shih said the parent perspective was missing from previous research. Preliminary findings showed that 33 percent of caregivers reported difficulties or delays in accessing care for their children because of cost; 24 percent of caregivers reported traveling more than 100 kilometers to receive a diagnosis for their child; and 21 percent of children ages 5 and older were not enrolled in school. The final report for this study is forthcoming.

Shih stated the existence of this network reflects an awareness and political will to provide for individuals with autism, but there is more

[1] Andy Shih is the senior vice president of scientific affairs at Autism Speaks in the United States.

work to be done. Although many countries have inclusive laws and policies on paper, in practice, children with developmental delays, behavioral disorders, or disabilities are often excluded from mainstream education, he said. Shih credited this contrast to a gap between policy and implementation. He emphasized the importance of recognizing that children with disabilities are children first—their disability is not their identity. Shih underscored that it is therefore critical to include children in the existing system, particularly in the context of the United Nations Sustainable Development Goals (UN SDGs).

SPECIAL NEEDS, SPECIAL RIGHTS

Donald Wertlieb warned participants about the misleading notion of "margins,"[2] stating that children with developmental delays and disabilities can be anywhere from 5 to 40 percent of a country's population. A conservative estimate of 20 percent is still a large "margin," he said, indicating that these children should be more prominently included in global efforts to build healthy, prosperous societies. He also shared his interest in connecting the dots between the United Nations Convention on the Rights of the Child (UN CRC) and the United Nations Convention on the Rights of Persons with Disabilities (UN CRPD), and suggested that a comparison of the UN SDGs, the UN CRC, and the UN CRPD would be an extremely valuable undertaking.

Wertlieb stated that the world is at a tipping point, with numerous reports and policies elevating the visibility of children with disabilities (see Box 5-1); at the same time, he pondered what children gain or lose by being on a "laundry list" of vulnerable or marginalized populations.

Wertlieb highlighted four transformative trends. First, he noted the growing number of children living with disabilities. Overall, these children make up between 5 and 25 percent of a country's population. According to UNICEF's State of the World's Children report released in 2013, 93 million children worldwide are living with disabilities (UNICEF, 2013). Wertlieb celebrated the progress made in reducing child mortality, but he urged researchers and decision makers to acknowledge new morbidity. With increased infant survival, he said, many children have disabilities that threaten to compromise their health and functioning. Second, he discussed a shift from medical models to bio-psycho-socio-cultural models. Third, a movement from narrow deficit models to holistic, ecological models that embrace strengths, as well as promotive and protective factors. Lastly, he discussed replacing charity-based approaches with

[2] Donald Wertlieb works with the Partnership for Early Childhood Development and Disability Rights and is based in the United States.

BOX 5-1
Reports and Policies Elevating the Visibility of Children with Disabilities

- UN CRC
- UN CRPD
- UN SDGs
- Incheon Declaration—*Education for 2030: Towards Inclusive and Equitable Quality Education and Lifelong Learning for All* (World Bank, 2015)
- A new policy in the United States on including children with disabilities in early childhood programs (HHS and ED, 2016)
- European Agency for Special Needs and Inclusive Education's launch of the Early Childhood Education project that assesses the interface between early childhood interventions and primary education, and builds on the agency's projects from 2004 and 2010[a]
- UNESCO (United Nations Educational, Scientific and Cultural Organization) has launched eLeSI—e-Learning for Social Inclusion, with modules for children ages 0 to 3 and 4 to 16[b]
- UNICEF will release Inclusive Early Childhood Development Guidance (UNICEF, 2014)

[a] See https://www.european-agency.org/agency-projects/inclusive-early-childhood-education (accessed March 1, 2016).
[b] See http://www.elesi.eu/index.php?lang=en (accessed March 1, 2016).
SOURCE: Wertlieb, 2015.

rights-based frameworks. On this last point, he said there is "less focus on handouts and more attention to 'hand-ups,'" as a way to cultivate human capital and invest in a stronger society.

Wertlieb and Vibha Krishnamurthy outlined a path to achieving the UN SDGs that includes cross-sectoral integration, collaboration and interoperability, and triple twin tracking.[3] Based on her work in Mumbai, India, Krishnamurthy stated that when disability is presented to communities as a special issue that care providers must face, they are usually overwhelmed. However, when framing the conversation by saying children with and without disabilities both benefit from early screenings and intervention, the task is perceived as less daunting.

Twin-track I, "mainstreaming," involves harmonizing disability policies and services with universal services and policies. According to

[3] Vibha Krishnamurthy is founder and director of the Ummeed Child Development Center in Mumbai, India.

Krishnamurthy, this means placing children with disabilities in the context of child development in general while ensuring practitioners provide the special services they need. In the Ummeed Center's Early Childhood Development and Disability Program, practitioners do this by training health workers to promote early child development in families and communities, detect delays and disabilities as early as possible, and provide referrals to specialized services such as hearing tests and wheelchair providers.

To describe twin-track II, coordinating child/family-centered and community-based care, Krishnamurthy reinforced the trend of moving from a deficit-based approach to a strengths-based approach and read a quote from *Poor Economics* (Banerjee and Duflo, 2011):

> The way the poor make decisions, at some level, is not that different from our own. They are no less rational or sophisticated than anyone else, and they are well aware that mistakes for them are costlier.

For her, it is critical for researchers and decision makers to realize that families are the experts in their own lives and that they will ultimately make a difference in their communities. This is an important consideration when building capacity for low- and middle-income countries (LMICs), she said.

Krishnamurthy then described twin-track III, integrating special knowledge of children from birth to age 3 with more traditional knowledge of older children and adults. She stated that this track should transfer the knowledge researchers have on young children to the education setting, as well as to young adults, as a way to help with the transition out of childhood to adulthood. Improving the lives of the most vulnerable people in society will make things better for everyone, she said. Krishnamurthy recommended looking past survival toward developmental outcomes, and building capacity in LMICs with an emphasis on family-centered and strengths-based approaches.

EARLY CHILDHOOD INTERVENTION: GLOBAL SURVEY RESULTS

Hollie Hix-Small defined early childhood interventions (ECIs) as interventions for children ages 0 to 3 or 5 who are living with disabilities or developmental delays,[4] are malnourished, have low birth weight, or have chronic illnesses. These interventions are also provided to children

[4] Hollie Hix-Small is an assistant professor at Portland State University and an ECI consultant from the United States.

who are at increased risk for delay due to family status, live in conflict or are displaced, or live in extreme poverty. She stated that numerous professionals and paraprofessionals provide ECI services to these children that are individualized, intensive, family centered, team based, evidence informed, outcome driven, and contextualized. Hix-Small said that the bedrock of ECI is having a team around the child. In the best models, the early interventionist takes a lead role and is supported by professionals from other disciplines, she said. The early interventionist works with the family within an ecological context and receives support from physical therapists, nutritionists, and speech and language pathologists, among other specialists.

Hix-Small presented a global survey she conducted in partnership with Emily Vargas-Baron to understand the state of ECI around the world.[5] The exploratory study aimed to document ECI services around the world, identify regional differences in programming, and make recommendations for developing and strengthening ECI systems. The survey, a collaboration between Open Society Foundations–London and the International Society on Early Intervention, was administered between December 2013 and July 2014. Hix-Small said surveys were available in English and French with online and offline versions, and were composed of 38 questions (see Box 5-2).

Hix-Small and Vargas-Baron received surveys from 392 respondents across 99 countries, but they eliminated some submissions because a few countries misunderstood "early childhood intervention services" and instead responded in regard to early childhood development services. In the end, the sample contained 81 countries. Fifty-five percent of countries from Europe were represented, 40 percent from Asia, 25 percent each from Africa and the Americas, and 16 percent from Oceana, said Hix-Small. Results showed that of the 81 countries, ECI was a high priority for 16 percent, a moderate priority for 41 percent, a low priority for 26 percent, and not a priority at all for the remaining 17 percent of countries. Hix-Small said that, overall, Asian countries reported ECI as a lower priority than the average countries in other regions.[6]

Hix-Small presented a recommended developmental pathway for the creation of ECI services that starts with intersectorial collaboration and ends with phased expansion. This pathway, presented in full in Figure 5-1, draws on Vargas-Baron's extensive experience in developing ECI services. Additional recommendations for developing ECI services as prevented by Hix-Small are included in Box 5-3.

---

[5] Emily Vargas-Baron is director of the RISE Institute.

[6] Data are currently unpublished, but will soon be made available on the RISE Institute website: http://www.riseinstitute.org/about.htm (accessed March 1, 2016).

BOX 5-2
Survey Questions from Global Survey of ECI

Questions from the global survey assessed:

- Policy frameworks and regulations;
- Child identification, assessment, and program planning;
- Provision of quality ECI services;
- Program accountability and data-based decision making;
- Personnel training; and
- Financial support for ECI services.

Most questions could be answered with yes, no, or don't know.

SOURCE: Hix-Small, 2015.

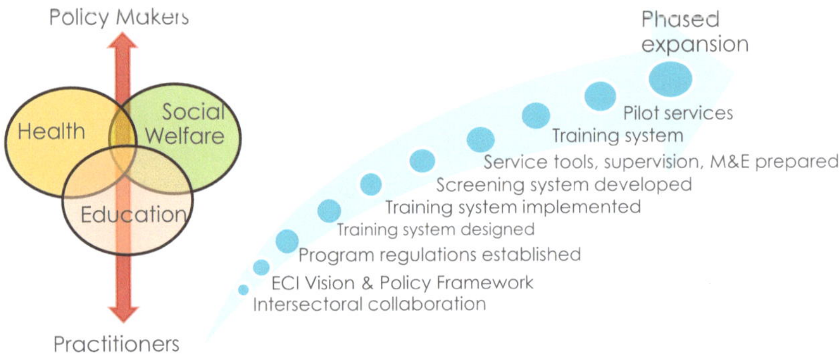
Policy Makers
Health
Social Welfare
Education
Practitioners
Phased expansion
Pilot services
Training system
Service tools, supervision, M&E prepared
Screening system developed
Training system implemented
Training system designed
Program regulations established
ECI Vision & Policy Framework
Intersectoral collaboration

FIGURE 5-1 ECI developmental pathway.
NOTE: ECI = early childhood intervention; M&E = monitoring and evaluation.
SOURCE: Hix-Small, 2015.

Key messages from the survey as reported by Hix-Small include that several countries are developing broad and strong ECI foundations but that international, regional, and national support is needed to develop sustainable systems. She also said that countries have differing priorities and starting points, so culturally and contextually relevant examples from policy to practice are needed.

BOX 5-3
Recommendations for Developing ECI Services

- Global, regional, and national advocacy campaigns
- National policy and strategic planning support
- National program guides and standards
- National screening and referral system
- Personnel development and standards
- Comparative financing studies
- Technical support

SOURCE: Hix-Small, 2015.

POLICY AND PROGRAM PERSPECTIVES FROM ALBANIA

Ariel Como discussed the national context for children with developmental delays, disabilities, and mental health issues in Albania.[7] According to Como, Albania has a population of almost 3 million people, one-fifth of whom are children under the age of 14. While reports may indicate that Albania has a set of laws governing policy and service delivery for all children, Como stated that an enabling environment for early childhood development has not been streamlined. He said that limited mechanisms are in place to coordinate across sectors to provide services for the holistic development of children under the age of 6 years. Examining mental health more broadly, Como stated that Albania has very few mental health professionals and a high number of people in institutions. He reasoned that so many people are in institutionalized care because of a lack of community services. He finished by stating that challenges for Albania include scaling services, building capacity, a lack of guidance on what practices to implement, and research gaps.

Liri Berisha described her work with the Albanian Children's Foundation (ACF).[8] Founded in 1996, the ACF has provided services to children with autism since 2006. In 2006, there were very few services available for children with autism, and according to Berisha, stigma was rampant in Albanian society. Moreover, families were burdened by caring for children with autism without any training or support from the state. Berisha

[7] Ariel Como is the national coordinator of Albania for the SEAN network and is an advisor to the Albanian Ministry of Health.

[8] Liri Berisha is president of the Albanian Children's Foundation (ACF) and former first lady of Albania.

said that the ACF focuses on early assessment and intervention services for children up to 14 years old. Two regional centers for autism provide treatment for children with autism and trainings for young professional therapists and those working with children in health care or educational facilities. Since inception, the ACF holds yearly intensive autism awareness campaigns spearheaded by parents of children with autism. In addition to training service providers, the organization publishes instructional materials and offers a 6-hour training guide for parents to care for their children and promote optimal development.

Berisha credits the ACF's success to several factors, starting with their partnership and coordination with parents, who are involved in each step of the organization's processes. Additionally, the ACF has a high standard of quality comparable to models in developing countries, she said. Thirdly, Berisha highlighted the organization's transparent fundraising mechanism and openness to the community, which have spurred donations. The ACF also works in close collaboration with pediatricians, teachers, and psychologists to enhance knowledge, training, and high-quality publications, stated Berisha. Finally, she attributed the ACF's high impact to the organization's dedication to data and research to inform their work.

POLICY AND RESEARCH PERSPECTIVES FROM MACEDONIA

Lidija Krstevska Dojcinovska discussed the laws and policies for children with disabilities in Macedonia across the areas of education, social protection, and health care. According to Dojcinovska, while there is no specific law on inclusive education in Macedonia, existing laws contain the principles that support it. The Law on Primary Education (2007) provides the right for children with developmental delays and disabilities to enroll in mainstream education or attend special schools. Prior to this law in 2008, children with these needs had to be enrolled in special schools. The National Strategy for the Development of Education 2005–2015 (The Parliament of the Republic of Macedonia, 2004) aimed to reduce discrimination in schools and increase support for children with disabilities in mainstream schools, as did the 2008 National Strategy for Deinstitutionalization (Government of FYR Macedonia, 2008). The National Strategy for Equalization of the Rights of People with Disabilities of 2010–2018 mandates the employment of special educators in mainstream schools along with continuous teacher training (Government of FYR Macedonia, 2010). Dojcinovska said that every document states that children with disabilities have (1) the same right to quality education as children without disabilities; (2) the right to choose and have an inclusive environment; and (3) are entitled to specific resources and expertise to satisfy their educational needs. Yet, these policies have not been translated on the ground, said Dojcinovska. While the legal framework for inclusive education is clear, there are not enough support systems for teachers and children with disabilities. Moreover, teachers do not receive enough training to work with these special needs students, and there is insufficient funding to develop services at the central and local levels.

In terms of health care and social protection, Dojcinovska said that laws in Macedonia provide for the early identification of children with disabilities, but that the country does not have an adequate strategy for early intervention. She did note that Macedonia has centers for social work; development counseling offices to monitor children born at risk of developing a developmental delay or disability; and speech therapists, psychologists, and physical therapists to diagnose and treat certain conditions. Dojcinovska stated that Macedonia faces several challenges including the early identification of delays and disabilities, which often occurs very late, and is unaccompanied by support services. Parents also avoid screenings so their child is not labeled, said Dojcinovska. There are challenges in the diagnostic and treatment process as well, she explained, where there is still limited knowledge about the treatment of some conditions such as autism, and professionals sometimes resort to disease classification rather than needs assessment. Finally, she said that more financial resources are needed for family support and the development of services at the local level.

Tatjana Zorcec presented preliminary results from the SEAN Caregiver Needs Study in Macedonia.[9] She said that the most alarming finding was that more than 60 percent of children with autism in Macedonia are nonverbal or minimally verbal (use single words only). Another finding was that parents received most information about autism from the Internet rather than their child's doctor, teacher, or other parents of children with autism, and that caring for these children puts significant financial strain on families as they pay for most services out of pocket. According to Zorcec, Macedonia has experienced a rapid increase in the number of children with autism, and there are insufficient resources available to support these children and their families. Yet there are some positive aspects in this situation, said Zorcec, including raised awareness about autism, some inclusion of children with autism in mainstream education, and plans to open a center for autism diagnosis.

POLICY PERSPECTIVE FROM GEORGIA

Maia Buchukuri highlighted Georgia's transition from institutionalization to social integration of children with special needs.[10] Buchukuri

---

[9] Tatjana Zorcec is the national coordinator for Autism for Macedonia.

[10] Maia Buchukuri is head of the Social Program Division, Ministry of Labor, Health, and Social Affairs in Georgia.

stated that of Georgia's population of 4 million, there are 10,000 children with disabilities and nearly 25,000 orphans.[11] The approach to child care reform in the country involved deinstitutionalization and reductions in abandonment via the development of alternative care and family support services. According to Buchukuri, several large institutions were closed from 2004 to 2015, resulting in a reduction in the number of children in institutionalized care from 5,500 to 200.

The ECI model in Georgia is interdisciplinary and multisectorial, said Buchukuri. The main pillars of the model are early detection, surveillance, and referral. Early childhood education and ECI are managed by the Ministry of Labor, Health, and Social Affairs, and the transition to preschool institutions and educational services is spearheaded by the Ministry of Science and Education. Buchukuri highlighted several successes including the development and implementation of several ECI services in the capital, Tbilisi, and other regions of Georgia. She also indicated Georgia has a sustainable funding system and a joint vision from several ministries regarding early child development, which has resulted in an annual increase in the number of children involved in ECI programs.

A REGIONAL PERSPECTIVE ON PREVENTION

Bettina Schwethelm provided UNICEF's strategies to address the complex needs of children with developmental delays and disabilities in Central and Eastern Europe and the Commonwealth of Independent States (CEE/CIS)[12]:

- Use home visiting services for the prevention, early identification, referral, and support to families of special needs children.
- Introduce developmental pediatrics to strengthen family-centered assessment and intervention.
- Promote social inclusion and learning in preschool settings.
- Advocate nationally for greater social inclusion.

Through the home visiting program that began in the region in 2011, Schwethelm said UNICEF is promoting the idea of comprehensive development of all young children and a continuum of care through ongoing case management, as presented by Krishnamurthy, Hix-Small, and Wertlieb. Content for the program is steeped in early child develop-

[11] See http://ssa.gov.ge/index.php?lang_id=ENG&sec_id=610 (accessed March 1, 2016).

[12] Bettina Schwethelm is an independent senior consultant who provides technical advice and guidance to the Young Child Health and Wellbeing program of the UNICEF Regional Office for CEE/CIS.

ment, prioritizes the prevention of developmental difficulties, and provides links to services, she said. To strengthen home visitor capacity, UNICEF, in partnership with the International Step by Step Association, developed regional guidance as well as 14 resource modules. Modules focus on developmental difficulties, attachment, stigma and discrimination, cross-sectorial coordination, and child maltreatment, among others. Schwethelm stated that the home visiting service has been evaluated in Bosnia and Herzegovina and results showed a positive effect on child outcomes and parent–child relationships (Yousafzai and Rasheed, 2015).

In 2013–2014, UNICEF mapped the available ECI resources in CEE/CIS across 21 countries and found that quality early identification and intervention was lacking in many countries (Ertem, 2015). Together with the Developmental Pediatrics Department of Ankara University, UNICEF has provided orientation training on developmental pediatrics and family-centered services and continued support to professionals in 10 countries of the region.

BREAKOUT SESSION ON CHILDREN WITH DEVELOPMENTAL DELAYS AND DISABILITIES

Shih summarized discussions from the breakout group on children with developmental delays and disabilities. In this breakout group, participants heard from Mariana Nikolova, another representative of the Karin Dom Foundation in Bulgaria. According to her, oftentimes governments or funders provide financial support for programs without forethought on how to continue services. For example, she said that in one area, funds were provided to train support personnel and therapists, but there was no job security for them once trained. After 3 months, they had to leave their positions. This reality disincentivizes prospective participants, she said. Another participant discussed World Bank investments and how money from the bank is given to local governments for disbursement. Yet there is no agreement within the government in terms of how to allocate resources to engender the outcomes intended by the funders.

During the discussion, Shih said participants highlighted how definitions of early childhood intervention and disability may vary, underscoring the need for a greater understanding of context for programming. Part of the context to be considered includes leadership, evaluation, and center- versus family-based models of intervention. Participants discussed the need for vertical and horizontal alignment of leadership requiring top-down or bottom-up approaches as well as cross-sector transfers of skills and lessons learned. Some participants noted that oftentimes programs and services do not have a built-in evaluation component. These participants remarked that strategic planners are removed from realities on the ground and are not informed about the challenges families face on a daily basis. Finally, several participants thought a center-based model would not reach all children living in families. Instead, a few participants said implementers should consider a community-based, capacity-building approach as they can be more cost-effective, encourage commitment at all levels as well as local ownership of programs, and empower families and community stakeholders.

6

Refugee, Immigrant, and Migrant Children

Returning to what Wertlieb referred to as the misleading notion of "margins," Joan Lombardi said that if one adds up all of the children at the margins, they become the central focus.[1] According to data from the European Commission, of the several hundred thousand refugees seeking asylum in the European Union, one in four are children. Lombardi described these children as those who have experienced violent conflicts, economic hardships, and forced migrations, sometimes traveling without their families. In addition, thousands of unaccompanied children are trafficked into and throughout the European Union. These vulnerable children form a diverse group in terms of culture, language, religion, and educational background. For Lombardi, there is a clear framework to provide refugee children with education and early childhood services. She encouraged workshop participants to take action to address the current Syrian crisis and other crises that hundreds of thousands of children face around the world.

A GLOBAL VIEW OF FORCIBLY DISPLACED PERSONS WORLDWIDE

Eskinder Negash presented a global picture of forcibly displaced people worldwide,[2] a number which is at its highest point since World

[1] Joan Lombardi is a senior advisor to the Bernard van Leer Foundation and based in the United States.

[2] Eskinder Negash is senior vice president for global engagement with the U.S. Committee for Refugees and Immigrants.

War II. He began by providing definitions of internally displaced persons, asylum seekers, and unaccompanied and separated minors.

- Refugee: Someone outside his or her country of nationality who is unable or unwilling to return because of persecution or a well-founded fear of persecution on account of race, religion, nationality, membership in a particular social group, or a political opinion (UN General Assembly, 1951)
- Internally displaced person: Someone who has been forcibly uprooted and displaced within their own country (UNHCR, 2015a)
- Asylum seeker: Someone who has applied for refugee status and is awaiting a determination of status (UNESCO, 2016)
- Unaccompanied and separated minor: Unaccompanied children under the age of 18 who have been separated from both parents or legal caregivers and are not being cared for by an adult (International Committee of the Red Cross et al., 2004).

In 2014, the United Nations High Commissioner for Refugees (UNHCR) reported 19.5 million refugees, 38.2 million internally displaced persons, and 1.8 million asylum seekers around the world (UNHCR, 2015a). Of the refugees, 51 percent were under age 18—children, as defined by international law—who are vulnerable, dependent, and developing (UNHCR, 2015a). At the end of 2014, Syria was the largest source of refugees (4.6 million; overtaking Afghanistan who had held the position for 3 decades) and reported 7.6 million internally displaced persons, the highest figure in the world (UNHCR, 2015a). Of the nearly 4.6 million current Syrian refugees, slightly more than half are children (UNHCR, n.d.).

Negash pointed out that although the current focus is on the conflict in Syria, millions of people are internally displaced or remain in protracted refugee situations. According to UNHCR, as of 2014, the five countries of origin for most refugees seeking resettlement are Syria, the Democratic Republic of the Congo, Myanmar, Iraq, and Somalia (UNHCR, 2015b). In sub-Saharan Africa alone, there were 3.7 million refugees at the end of 2014 (UNHCR, 2014). The countries from which the majority of refugees in Africa originate are the Democratic Republic of the Congo (53 percent), Somalia (23 percent), Eritrea (8 percent), Burundi (3 percent), and Sudan (3 percent). Dadaab, in northern Kenya near Somalia's border, is the world's largest refugee camp. Pakistan and Iran host nearly all 2.6 million Afghan refugees who have been living outside of Afghanistan for 30 years (UNHCR, 2014).

To address the high number of refugees and displaced children, Negash recommended recognizing displacement caused by gang violence and sexual orientation prejudice, as well as developing policies to grant "child protective status," which prevents the movement of children for the duration of the designation. He also suggested strengthening and creating uniformity in regional and national frameworks that include child-welfare standards to ensure protection. He encouraged UNHCR to work with additional resettlement countries to build capacity to receive new refugees. Finally, he recommended that the U.S. government prioritize raising the number of unaccompanied refugee minors accepted into the country. For Negash, this is the crisis of our time and encouraged workshop participants to take action.

THE MOTHER CHILD EDUCATION FOUNDATION, TURKEY: WORKING ACROSS RESEARCH, PRACTICE, AND POLICY

Suna Hanoz described the Mother Child Education Foundation's (ACEV's) efforts to provide educational programs and services to under-resourced populations.[3] According to Hanoz, ACEV was founded in 1993 in Turkey and performs research, develops and implements programs,[4] and creates policy. As the education system is very centralized in Turkey, she explained that ACEV partners with the ministries of education, agriculture, and family and social affairs to implement their programs. Through ACEV's programs, 900,000 children, parents, and illiterate adults have benefited from services offered via 11,000 trained professionals and paraprofessionals.

ACEV offers a 10-week intensive preschool and family support program for the marginalized Kurdish population living in underdeveloped regions of southeastern Turkey. According to Hanoz, this population typically has a low socioeconomic status. This group is also deprived of early childhood education services owing to the scarcity of such services in the region. She said this group faces challenges with language, as well. The majority of the children speak Kurdish at home, but school curricula are taught in Turkish. The ACEV program is implemented over the summer, in Ministry of Education schools. Trainers administer a paired curriculum for mothers and their children, aimed at 6-year-old children who have previously not received any early development services. The program aims to prepare children for entry into first grade in Turkish public schools. Simultaneously, trainers equip mothers with knowledge and skills to support their child's development. Hanoz said an evaluation of the program shows that children have enhanced cognitive, linguistic, physical, and socioemotional development and are better prepared for school compared to control groups that did not attend the program

---

[3] Suna Hanoz is a senior specialist with the Mother Child Education Foundation (ACEV).

[4] In addition to Turkey, ACEV works in Brazil, Germany, Laos, Lebanon, and Saudi Arabia.

(Bekman et al., 2011). Moreover, through the Mother Support Program, mothers in the program have increased awareness, knowledge, and skills related to child development and have decreased negative disciplining methods.

Since 2011, ACEV has implemented a 25-week Mother–Child Education Program with Palestinian refugees in long-term settlement camps in Beirut, Lebanon, in partnership with the Arab Resource Collective. The program teaches mothers to effectively interact with their preschool-aged children (4 to 6 years old). According to Hanoz, this program explores the extent to which early mother–child education programs can promote peaceful societies through building peaceful families and compassionate communities. Evaluations of this program show children's acquisition of socioemotional skills, executive function, and cognitive development, and mothers' improved patterns of parenting through responsiveness to children and less harsh discipline (Oweini and Issa, 2015).

ACEV plans to implement these programs with Syrian families in the future, as at the end of 2015, Turkey was home to 2.5 million Syrian refugees, half of which were under the age of 18. Importantly, 1.7 million of those refugees are not in camps. Rather, they are spread throughout Turkey. Early on when Turkey opened its borders to refugees, the government was slow to develop effective cooperation, said Hanoz. As time progressed and officials realized refugees were not likely to return home, relations between the government and nongovernmental organizations (NGOs) improved. Nevertheless, she said, many challenges remain, including that 70 percent of Syrian children are out of school and Syrians cannot work legally in Turkey. Hanoz indicated that there are inadequate resources to support Syrian refugees for short stays or long-term harmonization, and there are rising tensions between Turks and Syrians. To address these obstacles, Hanoz recommended working with families to build resilience and harmony within the family unit, providing children with the tools necessary to succeed, and learning as much from the current situation as possible to improve responses to and prevent future crises.

CHILD MIGRANTS IN THE UNITED STATES—AN ADVOCACY PERSPECTIVE

Human Rights Watch (HRW) investigates and documents human rights abuses in 90 countries, exposes findings to the media, and advocates for policy change. Alison Parker highlighted the human rights concerns facing four categories of migrants in the United States[5]: (1) unaccom-

[5] Alison Parker is director of Human Rights Watch's programs in the United States.

panied child migrants, (2) families separated across the United States–Mexico border, (3) children migrating with family members, and (4) child migrant workers. According to Parker, unaccompanied child migrants in the United States generally arrive via the United States–Mexico border, arriving from Mexico and Central America. She stated that 41,000 unaccompanied child migrants arrived in the United States in 2015 (Gordon, 2015). This vulnerable group has endured sexual violence; trafficking; involvement with criminal groups (gangs); lack of access to food, water, shelter, and education; and fear for their lives, according to Parker. For HRW, Parker said the greatest concern is that United States law does not require border authorities to consider the best interests of the children in their custody.

Parker stated that every day, families are separated across the United States–Mexico border. United States citizen children remain in the United States, and their undocumented parents are deported back to Mexico or Central America. Parker said there are 4.1 million United States citizen children who have undocumented parents living in the United States (Dwyer, 2014). She pointed out that these parents are constantly at risk of deportation and are faced with the difficult decision of returning to their birth country, a place no one in the family has connections to, or to agree to be deported without their children. If they are deported, parents generally try several times to cross the border to be reunited with their United States citizen children, Parker said. Children facing family separation often face increased levels of anxiety and psychological harm. In addition, the well-being of these children is worsened by the limited resources of family members who have taken them in; these children often perform poorly in school, as well (Urban Institute, 2004).

Many children traveling with their parents to the United States from Mexico are first held in Border Patrol facilities, said Parker. Through their work with families, HRW has heard countless stories of freezing temperatures and insufficient food in the facilities leading to illness. Afterward, families are sent to detention centers for several weeks and are sometimes separated from one another in different family detention facilities across the country. These families suffer from premigration trauma, psychological and health consequences from the hostile conditions of detention centers, and several have attempted suicide (Pilkington, 2015a,b). Parker said that through HRW's advocacy, the average duration of family detention has reduced (Human Rights Watch, 2015; Preston, 2015).

According to Parker, the United States has between 300,000 and 800,000 children working in the agricultural industry (National Center for Farmworker Health, 2012). Although child labor is outlawed in the country, there is a major exception for farm work, she said. Children as young as 7 years old have shared stories with HRW about picking strawberries in Florida, shucking peas in Virginia, and hoeing cotton in Texas. These children have dropped out of school, incurred injuries from farm equipment, have been exposed to pesticides, and endured physical abuse, Parker said.

Parker closed by offering some suggestions and lessons drawn from her experience working with the many types of migrants within the United States. She called on workshop participants to do the following:

- Recognize children can experience trauma before, during, and after migration.
- Examine the reception of children and their families at the border.
- Embrace the best interests of children when creating policies.
- Keep families and children together.
- Prohibit the detention of child migrants as a means of migration control.
- Prohibit the employment of children.
- Recognize that some child migrants are victims of criminal organizations around the world.
- Provide holistic services—health, legal, and social—to migrant children and families.

THE TRANSATLANTIC FORUM ON INCLUSIVE EARLY YEARS

Jan Peeters presented the work of the Transatlantic Forum on Inclusive Early Years,[6,7] which was organized by the Centre for Innovation in the Early Years and the Migration Policy Institute, with support of the King Baudouin Foundation and 10 foundations from Europe and the United States. The forum, composed of 120 policy makers from the United States and Europe and 110 leading researchers from around the world, convened seven times between 2013 and 2016 to discuss relevant issues in early childhood education and care, focusing on children from low-income, refugee, and migrant families (Peeters and Vandekerckhove, 2015). Meetings covered such topics as

- Access to early childhood services;
- Curriculum innovation and workforce preparation;

---

[6] Jan Peeters is coordinator of the Centre for Innovation in the Early Years at the Research Centre for ECEC (VBJK) at Ghent University in Belgium.

[7] For more information on the Transatlantic Forum on Inclusive Early Years, please visit http://www.europe-kbf.eu/en/projects/early-childhood/transatlantic-forum-on-inclusive-early-years (accessed April 1, 2016).

- Parent engagement; monitoring and evaluation;
- Integrated systems and effective transitions in early childhood; and
- Multilingualism and multiple identities/belonging.

Access to early childhood services was an important topic for the forum, Peeters remarked. He said that accessibility, affordability, and availability are just as important considerations for high-quality services as desirability, usefulness, and meaningfulness to migrant families. During the Forum he also stated that clear arguments for the benefits of these services are necessary to convince parents to use services (Vandenbroeck and Lazzari, 2014). As discussed during the Forum, Peeters said that the real problem is it is not hard to reach parents; it is hard to reach services.

Peeters researched workforce competencies that are necessary at the team and individual level when working with migrant and refugee children and children at risk (Peeters and Sharmahd, 2014). He recommended openness to dialogue with parents, colleagues, and children on the basis of reciprocity; an engagement and ability to work toward social change; the ability to reflect critically on one's own pedagogical practice and that of the team and the institution working in these hyperdiverse contexts; and the ability to create new pedagogical knowledge and practice.

Regarding parent engagement, Peeters said the Transatlantic Forum on Inclusive Early Years stated that there needs to be a shift toward "demand-led" services. Rather than requiring parents and children to adapt to available services, the forum encourages decision makers to engage in reciprocal relationships with migrant parents to cocreate programs and services that have meaning to migrant families. Also, in understanding that parent participation has different meanings in different contexts, Peeters encouraged workshop participants to see participation as more than just parents reading to their children, but having parents engaged in important decisions in early childhood centers that affect their children's lives.

In addressing the large number of refugees coming to Europe, the Forum emphasized the need for integrated systems, particularly in regard to how the educational sector, child protection sector, and health care systems should work together to ensure smooth transitions between home and early childhood education. Peeters said that school readiness does not mean that only the child is ready. Rather, children, families, schools, and communities all need to be prepared for the transition (Dumcius et al., 2014). He remarked that if parents—particularly parents of refugee children—are not familiar with the educational system, it is difficult for them to prepare their children for the next step. This is particularly true for families who speak languages other than what is taught in school.

BREAKOUT SESSION ON MIGRANT, IMMIGRANT, AND REFUGEE CHILDREN

Janna Patterson summarized the discussion from the breakout session on migrant, immigrant, and refugee children.[8] According to her, participants focused on best practices in the integration of services across sectors and engaging migrants in programming. Participants discussed one case from Chile in which a baby died after her family was denied health services because she was not registered in the system. The death of this baby led the government to establish offices for registration for unified services across health, education, nutrition, and other sectors, she said. One participant remarked that this registration system led to better capacity to address issues across stages of life.

Breakout session participants highlighted the Head Start program for migrants in the United States as well as the United States resettlement program, both of which have contributed to positive outcomes for migrants. Also, a few participants noted that Belgium places the United Nations Convention on the Rights of the Child above national law, which has benefitted migrants via increased funding for schools that serve migrant populations. In turn, schools see migrant students as a positive asset as they are tied to funding resources and also bring with them a diversity of experience that benefits the entire school.

To further engage migrants, participants said that in many areas, young migrants are becoming advocates for themselves. Participants cited the DREAM (Development, Relief, and Education for Alien Minors) movement in the United States as a prominent example. Some participants suggested combining data and personal stories to lift up migrant experiences and show positive examples of how immigrants hold prominent places in society and have strengthened the fabric of their new societies.

---

[8] Janna Patterson is a senior program officer, Maternal, Newborn, and Child Health, The Bill & Melinda Gates Foundation.

7

Combining the Science of Child Development with Quality Measurement to Support Early Childhood Programs and Policies

According to Abbie Raikes,[1] who provided the keynote talk, early childhood development has made its global debut in the United Nations Sustainable Development Goals (UN SDGs). Target 4.2 of UN SDG Goal 4 on education explicitly recognizes early childhood care and education as a necessary part of a child's holistic development and well-being.[2] Moving forward, it will be necessary to ensure understanding that development starts at birth, as well as ensuring the importance of integrating preprimary programs; parenting programs; and health, education, and nutrition programs, she said.

Raikes views measurement as an important element to track trends and investments at the population level. The question then becomes how to translate these components into feasible measurements at scale. Measurement can encourage developmentally informed practice by describing children's development at key transitions such as formal entry into school. It can also describe the link between context and outcomes, she said. Perhaps most importantly, Raikes emphasized how measurement holds stakeholders accountable for improving children's environments and development, and that measurement can promote equity. As pre-

[1] Abbie Raikes is the technical development lead for the Measuring Early Learning Quality and Outcomes Project at UNICEF.

[2] Target 4.2 states: "By 2030, ensure that all girls and boys have access to quality early childhood development, care and preprimary education so that they are ready for primary education." For more information, visit http://www.un.org/sustainabledevelopment/education (accessed April 1, 2016).

BOX 7-1
Principles for Consideration in the Development of Measurement Tools

- Ensure that all children are counted: Create measures for use across different settings and languages. For Raikes, this involves creating measures across all settings so children are captured wherever they are, from birth to age 8.
- Ensure all children's skills are acknowledged: Create culturally sensitive measures with an adequate range.
- Measure context: Include child development and their environments.
- Take action: Measurement is only worth investing in if it informs action on behalf of children.

SOURCE: Raikes, 2015.

sented in Box 7-1, Raikes offered several principles that should be considered when developing measurement tools.

Raikes presented two projects addressing the question of measurement at scale. The first is a project by the World Health Organization (WHO)—with support from the Bernard van Leer Foundation—to develop a set of global indicators for child development from birth to age 3. The WHO project will field test and recommend a set of indicators to assess child development at the population level across the 0 to 3 age group. The second project taking the issue of measurement at scale is the Measuring Early Learning and Quality Outcomes Project. This project is a collaboration between UNICEF, the United Nations Educational, Scientific and Cultural Organization (UNESCO), the World Bank, and the Brookings Institution, with support from the Children's Investment Fund Foundation and several other partners. Phase 1 of the project, "consensus to country action," has three goals: (1) convene expert groups on quality, child development, and learning; (2) develop and pretest two new tools (child development and learning, and quality) that are conceptually linked; and (3) conduct institutional assessments on scaling the assessment. Raikes noted that although two tools were developed from this project, the main goal was to create a method for defining a common core.

Looking to the future, Raikes provided three goals for using "collective measurement expertise." She said the first goal should be integrating measurement to put forth a vision for measurement for children from birth through age 8. Next, researchers should work to create systems of measurement with countries participating in more than one effort. Finally, she said that governments should partner with local or regional research hubs to improve measurement over time.

THE AGES AND STAGES QUESTIONNAIRE: INVENTORY

Hollie Hix-Small provided an overview of the Ages and Stages Questionnaire: Inventory (ASQ: I), a direct child assessment instrument that targets children ages 1 to 36 months and evaluates progress over time. This measure was developed from the Ages and Stages Questionnaire (ASQ) items in 2006 at the University of Oregon.[3] It has been studied in Kenya, Madagascar, Taiwan, and with indigenous populations in the United States, and is now available for wider research use, said Hix-Small.[4]

Hix-Small said that the ASQ and the ASQ: I vary in many ways. While the ASQ is a screening tool meant to identify children 1 to 66 months old who are at risk of having developmental delays or disabilities, the ASQ: I is a progress monitoring tool that is currently available for children ages 1 to 36 months. Because the ASQ: I offers a continuous measure with age-appropriate starting points, parents or evaluators can start with survey questions appropriate for the developmental stage of the child. Hix-Small noted that in this way, the ASQ: I offers more flexibility than the ASQ and accounts for special cases such as a 6-month-old who is functioning more like a 3-month-old.

According to Hix-Small, parents are very involved in the administration of the ASQ: I; they respond to questions from survey administrators about their children's progress and actively elicit skills from their children. She said that some workshop participants might think that parents in low- and middle-income countries cannot answer questions about their child's development in a reliable and valid manner, but emerging research suggests parents are more than capable of answering these questions (Abubakar et al., 2010). In fact, in Madagascar, Hix-Small said that parents have underreported their children's development.

Hix-Small said the ASQ items have been translated into more than 37 languages and can be administered in two formats—with items grouped by domain and items grouped by activities. She explained that it is possible to arrange culturally appropriate activities that are more authentic and natural for the child and to collect data through observation. Hix-Small also said that this tool has several policy implications. First, ASQ: I is a low-cost and change-sensitive way to monitor child outcomes. It is

---

[3] For more information on the Ages and Stages Questionnaire, please visit: http://agesandstages.com/products-services/asq3 (accessed April 4, 2016).

[4] An adapted version of the instrument was used in India, Indonesia, Peru, and Senegal (Fernald et al., 2012).

also a technically sound tool to monitor change across developmental domains, she noted. Hix-Small said program implementers can use the ASQ: I to improve programming, accountability to donors, and increase parent awareness of child outcomes. Finally, policy makers can use the tool as a more robust measure of child progress allowing for program comparisons on child outcomes. Looking ahead, Hix-Small recommended additional research in the following areas: administration methods in varying regional and cultural contexts; item "functioning" within and between populations; additional concurrent validity studies; and development of country-specific percentile ranges.

THE GUIDE FOR MONITORING CHILD DEVELOPMENT

Krishnamurthy presented the Guide for Monitoring Child Development (GMCD), a clinical, open-ended evaluation and intervention to enhance developmental monitoring, support, and management of developmental difficulties. This tool, which has been in development by Ilgi Ertem and colleagues at Ankara University in Turkey since 1995 (Ertem et al., 2008), aims to catalyze provider–caregiver partnerships, and advance approaches to early childhood development and developmental difficulties in health systems. Krishnamurthy said the tool addresses two barriers to accessing children in low- and middle-income countries (LMICs): a lack of caregiver training in early childhood development and a lack of internationally standardized tools. The GMCD, as outlined by Krishnamurthy, reflects a bioecological theory; monitors and supports, rather than screens; and identifies and addresses risk factors.

Krishnamurthy presented examples of the questions asked in the guide (see Box 7-2). The first question is the only closed question; the remain-

BOX 7-2
Questions Asked in the GMCD

Question 1: Caregiver concerns: Do you have any concerns about your child's development?

Question 2: Communication, expressive language: How does your child let you know when she wants something? What kinds of sounds and words does she use?

Question 8: Developmental support: What do you do to support your child's development? How do you play with her? How do you get her to communicate?

SOURCE: Krishnamurthy, 2015.

ing questions are open-ended and are aimed at generating a dialogue between the administrator and the parent. The guide is composed of 10 questions, the last 2 of which address maternal depression and other risk factors, instituting the "support" component of the guide. Krishnamurthy says that although the guide takes only 15 minutes to complete, in some instances, this is the first opportunity the caregiver has had to talk about her child's development. Many caregivers end the discussion feeling reassured that they can discuss their child's development with a health care provider, according to Krishnamurthy.

Krishnamurthy said that the International GMCD was completed in May 2015. Researchers worked in Argentina, India, South Africa, and Turkey for 5 years to determine if development in healthy children is similar in different countries and if these similarities can be used to develop an open-access international GMCD that does not require standardization.[5] More than 20,000 children enrolled over the course of 5 years and 3 phases (standardization for years 1–3; establishment of validity during years 3 and 4; and implementation, years 4 and 5). Based on preliminary analyses, findings showed that developmental milestones from age 0 to 42 months were attained at similar ages (by both sexes) in different countries by children without known health risks.

THE INTERNATIONAL DEVELOPMENT AND EARLY LEARNING ASSESSMENT

Ivelina Borisova presented Save the Children's International Development and Early Learning Assessment (IDELA),[6] a direct child assessment instrument that targets children aged 3.5 to 6.5 years (see Box 7-3). IDELA measures motor development, emergent language and literacy, emergent math/numeracy, and socioemotional development, as well as approaches to learning. According to Borisova, IDELA includes cross-cutting elements such as motivation, persistence at completing tasks, and self-regulation. The assessment takes 30 minutes to administer per child and includes 24 items across the four domains. To ensure that children do not feel like they are being assessed, tasks in IDELA are designed to be play based and interactive.

Flexibility is built into IDELA, said Borisova. The tool can be contextualized at the national level or regional level and can account for linguistic

[5] The International GMCD was developed in partnership between Ankara University, Centro Rosarino de Estudios Perinatales, Ummeed Child Development Center, University of Pretoria, and Yale University.

[6] At the time of the workshop, Ivelina Borisova was director, Early Childhood Development Impact and Innovations at Save the Children.

BOX 7-3
What Is IDELA?[a]

- A direct child assessment
- Intended for global use; feasible in low-income countries
- Successfully adapted and used in varied contexts—28 countries to date
- Monitors and tracks progress on a population or community level
- Tracks effect of interventions; compares effectiveness of approaches
- Intended to improve programs, policy, and practice and inspire investment

[a] For more information on IDELA, please visit: http://resourcecentre.savethechildren.se/library/international-development-and-early-learning-assessment-technical-paper (accessed April 4, 2016).
SOURCE: Borisova, 2015.

differences, depending on the country's level of diversity. Further, optional subscales accompany the core items. This means that countries making a big push on health and hygiene practices in preschool can add additional questions for this target, she said. Additionally, optional upward extensions can be added to many of the subscales to avoid "ceiling effects" in the more urban, middle-income, and highly developed populations. According to Borisova, countries can also add culturally or context-specific items to the core IDELA items. She said that to date, most countries take this option. In discussing adaptation of the tool, Borisova stated that Save the Children has a systematic process for introducing IDELA in new countries and has been successful in introducing a generic assessment into unique settings and making the tool work across diverse populations. In fact the tool has been used in 28 countries to date. She believes the flexibility IDELA offers is something that creates global linkages between countries and contexts while remaining a standardized tool for comparison.

Data collected through the administration of IDELA alongside a simple caregiver questionnaire can show disparities between children from various backgrounds. In Ethiopia for example, children from higher socioeconomic status have significantly higher literacy scores than counterparts with low socioeconomic status, 53 percent compared to 35 percent (Pisani et al., 2015). Similar disparities were found in skill variation in Bhutan for urban (40 percent) versus rural children (28 percent) (Dowd et al., under review) (see Figure 7-1).

In assessing skill variation in Mali, IDELA data showed that children with literate mothers scored higher than children with illiterate mothers

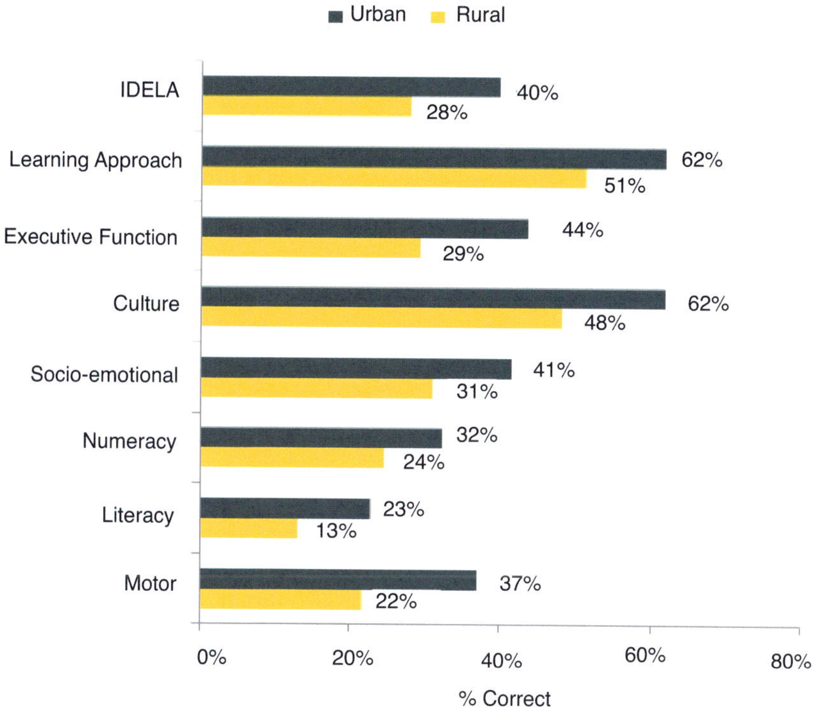

FIGURE 7-1 Skill variation by locality in Bhutan, 2015.
NOTE: IDELA = International Development and Early Learning Assessment.
SOURCE: National ECCD Impact Evaluation Study 2015, Save the Children Bhutan with the Ministry of Education of Bhutan, http://resourcecentre.savethechildren.se/library/national-eccd-impact-evaluation-study-2015 (accessed April 4, 2016).

in numeracy (42 percent compared to 34 percent) and socioemotional development (49 percent compared to 42 percent) (Thera et al., 2015).

Borisova also highlighted differences between children who have access to early childhood services and those who do not, and how these data can affect policy. Findings from IDELA show that in Ethiopia, children with access to high-quality early childhood programming have significant skill gains compared to children who receive standard programming offered through the government (39 percent gains compared to 10 percent gains) (Amente et al., 2013). Further, Borisova discussed the compounded disadvantage children can face on school readiness skills. In a national school readiness study in Bhutan, the difference in school readiness skills between children attending an early childhood development program and those who did not was, on average, only 6 percent

BOX 7-4
IDELA's Implications for Practice and Policy

- Deepening equity analyses globally; documenting what approaches close the equity gaps we see across and within countries
- Exploring effectiveness of different modes of delivery of early childhood development services
- Expanding partnerships and national use of the tool
- Longitudinal work looking at links between early learning and later school outcomes
- Making data and tools easily accessible to wider group of actors

SOURCE: Borisova, 2015.

(27 percent for early childhood development attendees versus 21 percent for nonattendees). However, when an added factor was added, such as socioeconomic status, the gap in skills widened significantly, and children from low-income families not attending preschool scored almost 20 percentage points lower compared to peers from wealthier families attending preschool (Dowd et al., under review).

Borisova closed by discussing the need for multipartner engagement at the national level to make the best use of the tool and the data it can offer ministries and relevant stakeholders. She presented implications for practice and policy, as provided in Box 7-4.

THE VIOLENCE AGAINST CHILDREN SURVEYS AND THE THRIVES TECHNICAL PACKAGE

Ruth Perou presented the U.S. Centers for Disease Control and Prevention's (CDC's) Violence Against Children Surveys (VACS), nationally representative household surveys of children and young adults ages 13 to 24.[7] In addition to the surveys, which address topics such as gender attitudes, witnessing violence, violence perpetration, and health outcomes, the surveys are accompanied by a THRIVES technical package to protect children from violence and adversity (see Box 7-5).

According to Perou, despite that many countries are unaware of the extent of violence against their children, studies have shown that exposure to violence during childhood can increase vulnerability to a number

[7] Ruth Perou is a behavioral scientist at the U.S. Centers for Disease Control and Prevention.

BOX 7-5
THRIVES—A Global Technical Package to Help Protect Children from Trauma and Adversity

Training in parenting for caretakers
Household economic strengthening
Reduce violence by legislative protection
Improve services for victims of violence
Value norms that protect children
Educate and build life skills
Surveillance to monitor trends and progress

SOURCE: Hillis et al., 2015.

of mental and physical health problems such as depression, unwanted pregnancy, cardiovascular disease, diabetes, and human immunodeficiency virus (HIV). Perou said the VACS and accompanying technical package were developed to estimate the extent of violence around the world, stimulate prevention and response efforts, and monitor progress. To date, the CDC has implemented VACS in 16 countries, and demand from other countries has been very high, said Perou.

Perou presented the latest data from the VACS. Findings show that in eight VACS countries, 4 to 38 percent of girls and 6 to 21 percent of boys aged 18 to 24 experienced sexual violence prior to turning 18 (Sumner et al., 2015) (see Figure 7-2). In seven VACS countries, 42 to 66 percent of girls and 52 to 76 percent of boys experienced physical violence before age 18 (Sumner et al., 2015) (see Figure 7-3). Research also shows associations between exposure to childhood sexual violence and increased risk of negative health conditions and behavior such as HIV, sexually transmitted diseases, pregnancy complications, alcohol use, suicidal ideation, and depression (Reza et al., 2009). According to Perou, most individuals reporting physical or sexual violence did not receive services for their abuse (Sumner et al., 2015); very few ever sought services. This may be due to a lack of services, being unaware services exist, or stigma, according to Perou.

Findings from the VACS have provided data to help countries respond to physical and sexual abuse as well as develop and launch violence prevention programs, said Perou. The THRIVES technical package includes programs and policies that are effective in preventing violence. Country-level responses have included legislation; school-based curricula about violence; service provision strategies; and an increase in workforce capacity of clinicians, police, social workers, and teachers.

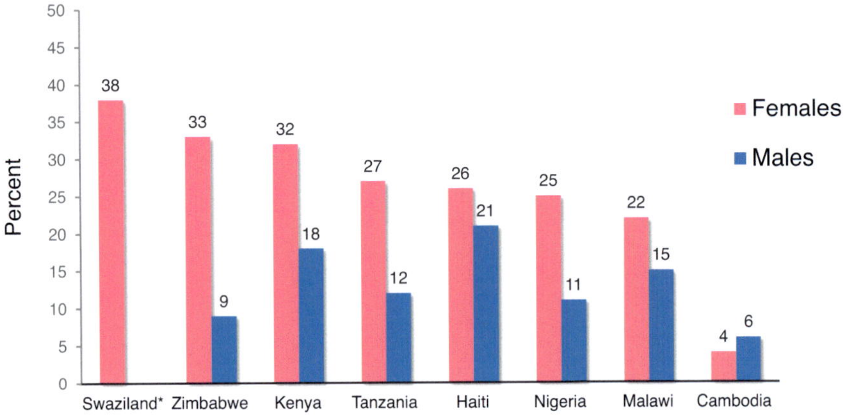

FIGURE 7-2 Prevalence of sexual violence prior to age 18 reported by females and males 18–24 years of age in eight VACS country sites.
* Only girls interviewed in Swaziland.
SOURCE: Sumner et al., 2015.

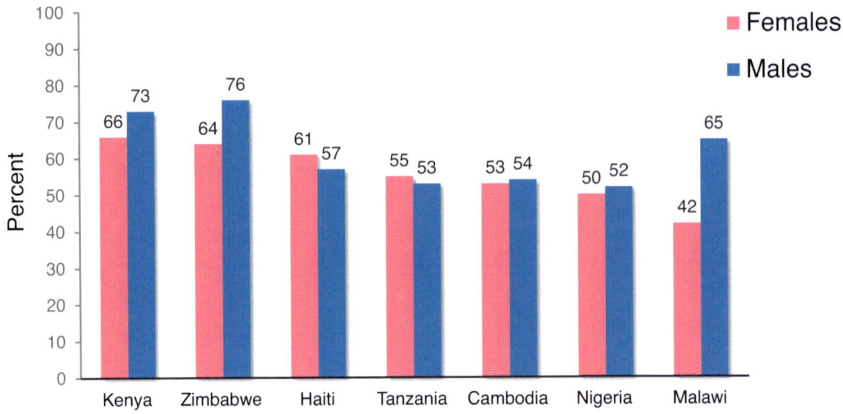

FIGURE 7-3 Prevalence of physical violence prior to age 18 reported by females and males 18–24 years of age by parents, adult caregivers, and authority figures in seven VACS country sites.
SOURCE: CDC, 2015.

A GLOBAL PERSPECTIVE ON MEASUREMENT: IMPLICATIONS FOR POLICY

Emily Vargas-Baron provided her perspective on early childhood policy and the various programmatic implications that accompany these policies in the era of the UN SDGs.[8] She believes some countries will try to achieve improved child development by using future measurement capacities of the UN SDGs. However, countries will likely create many additional indicators and targets that fit their national contexts. This will result in what Vargas-Baron referred to as a "patchwork quilt" of efforts around the world in which some countries follow the global indicators and their targets and others may not do so.

Vargas-Baron highlighted that many countries do have one or more policy instruments for early childhood development. At the time of the workshop, 75 countries had instruments, 10 more were reported to have them, and 23 were preparing them. Of these countries, Vargas-Barón said that 60 percent were LMICs. She did note that while many countries had instruments, not all of them included indicators, effectively making them more similar to "policy statements" than true national early childhood development policies or strategic plans. For those countries whose instruments include indicators, the indicators are predominantly operational or process indicators with inputs and outputs that are essential for policy implementation, said Vargas-Baron. According to a recent study, relatively few of the indicators used in early childhood development policies were outcome indicators, which is problematic (Vargas-Baron and Schipper, 2012). She said that it is critically important to develop a system to measure early childhood development outcomes and to use those outcomes for planning purposes.

While the United Nations Millennium Development Goals (UN MDGs) lacked an early childhood development goal, Vargas-Baron highlighted several UN SDGs that include targets related to early childhood development and early childhood intervention (see Box 7-6 for a full list). She said that these targets provide an opportunity to establish early childhood development and early childhood intervention indicators, noting that while this likely will not be achieved in the first round of indicators, specialists working on the UN MDGs took 4 years to complete and adopt their full list of indicators for use around the world.

Vargas-Baron summarized what she believes to be several key issues. First, she said that early childhood learning is not the same as early childhood development; learning is a subset of development, and researchers and decision makers need to take a broader view of child development.

[8] Emily Vargas-Baron is director of the RISE Institute in the United States.

BOX 7-6
UN SDG Goals and Targets That Incorporate Early Childhood Development and Early Childhood Interventions

- Poverty: 1.2 (young children living in poverty), 1.3 and 1.4 (services for children living in poverty), 1.5 (resources)
- Nutrition and food security: 2.1 (end hunger; access to food), 2.2 (end malnutrition, mothers and infants, stunting, etc.)
- Health and well-being: 3.2 (reduce neonatal and child mortality), 3.8 (universal health coverage and services)
- Education: 4.2 (early childhood development), 4.5 (equity), 4a (learning environments), 4c (qualified teachers)
- Gender: 5.2 (gender-based violence against women and children)
- Water and sanitation: 6.1 (drinkable water), 6.2 (good sanitation)
- Reduce inequality within and between nations: 10.2 (child rights)
- Safe, resilient, and sustainable settlements: 11.7 (for women and children)
- Peaceful and inclusive societies: 16.2 (end child abuse), 16.9 (legal identity and birth registration)

SOURCE: http://www.un.org/sustainabledevelopment/sustainable-development-goals (accessed April 4, 2016).

For example, 1 to 2 years of preprimary education and school readiness is not all encompassing of child development, which includes child health, nutrition, sanitation, education, protection, and child rights. Second, she stated that of necessity, national, intracountry, regional, and municipal needs must come before international needs. Countries will vary in their relative emphasis on topics such as fragile birth status; malnutrition and chronic illness; disabilities; and high-risk status and child protection. She also said that in most countries where she has worked, countries are very interested in having good indicators and measures for child development, but sometimes they lack the requisite expertise to develop them. Vargas-Baron said that countries further along in using effective measures might offer technical assistance to set indicators, measures, and targets, and validate instruments.

Vargas-Baron noted some challenges moving forward. She said that early childhood development and early childhood intervention specialists will need to include early childhood and marginalized populations in the development of UN SDG indices such as the social progress index, the People's Report Card, and others. Such efforts rarely include early childhood development in their international indices.

Additionally, she said that policy makers and policy researchers should be invited to participate in the development of indicators to offer nations guidance in developing national UN SDG plans. To offer this guidance, Vargas-Barón said a measurement research agenda should include population-level assessment of child development by age bands, parenting behaviors, assessment of the quality of early childhood development and early childhood intervention programs, and child equity.

CLOSING REMARKS

At the conclusion of the workshop, Liana Ghent remarked that the workshop provided a number of practical suggestions to bridge the gaps between research, policy, and practice.[9] For her, close cooperation and shared learning between these fields will promote cross-sectorial cooperation and coordination. She linked some messages from the workshop to the International Step by Step Assocation (ISSA) regional membership association that focuses on Europe and Central Asia. First, Ghent said the workshop has helped to inform ISSA's Early Childhood Workforce Initiative, a partnership with Results for Development, which targets competencies, standards, support for improvement, and empowering the early childhood workforce. Ghent emphasized that issues discussed in the workshop will continue to be explored in ISSA's Conference 2016[10]: Early Childhood in Times of Rapid Change, during which ideas will be taken further, including how to define meaningful learning during times of rapid change. According to Ghent, the iYCG Forum will benefit the global early childhood community if it continues to link to regional networks, as it did in its partnership with the ISSA and the Open Society Foundations for the workshop in Prague.

In her closing remarks, Klaus stated that one thread tied together all of the presentations relating to children at the margins: the importance of data in raising awareness and making inequality visible. She highlighted an Open Society Foundations report drawing attention to the lack of data on Roma entitled, *No Data—No Progress* (McDonald and Negrin, 2010). This report could have easily been called *No Data—No Problem*, she said, because for many, if they do not see a problem, it does not exist. She thanked presenters for demonstrating the myriad ways marginalization affects child development and for motivating participants to take action through scientific and programmatic developments.

---

[9] Liana Ghent is executive director of the ISSA.

[10] See http://www.issa.nl/content/save-date-issas-2016-conference (accessed April 4, 2016).

References

Abubakar, A., P. Holding, F. Van de Vijver, G. Bomu, and A. Van Baar. 2010. Developmental monitoring using caregiver reports in a resource-limited setting: The case of Kilifi, Kenya. *Acta Paediatrica* 99(2):291-297.

Adamson, P., J. Bradshaw, P. Hoelscher, and D. Richardson. 2007. *Child Poverty in Perspective: An overview of child well-being in rich countries.* (Innocenti Report Card). Florence, Italy: UNICEF Innocenti Research Centre.

Almas, A. N., K. A. Degnan, A. Radulescu, C. A. Nelson, C. H. Zeanah, and N. A. Fox. 2012. Effects of early intervention and the moderating effects of brain activity on institutionalized children's social skills at age 8. *Proceedings of the National Academy of Sciences of the United States of America* 109(Supplement 2):17228-17231.

Amente, A., A. Yenew, I. Borisova, and A. J. Dowd. 2013.*Emergent literacy and math (ELM) intervention endline report.* Fairfield, CT: Save the Children.

Atwoli, L., D. Ayuku, J. Hogan, J. Koech, R. Vreeman, S. Ayaya, P. Braitstein. 2014. Impact of domestic care environment on trauma and posttraumatic stress disorder among orphans in western Kenya. *PloS ONE* 9(3):e89937.

Banerjee, A. V., and E. Duflo. 2011. *Poor economics: A radical rethinking of the way to fight global poverty.* New York: PublicAffairs.

Bekman, S., A. Aksu-Koç, and E. Erguvanlı-Taylan. 2011. Effectiveness of an intervention program for six-year-olds: A summer-school model. *European Early Childhood Education Research Journal* 19(4):409-431.

Borisova, I. 2015. *Measuring development and early learning globally: The International Development and Early Learning Assessment (IDELA).* Presentation to the Forum on Investing in Young Children Globally. Prague, Czech Republic.

Bos, K. J., C. H. Zeanah, A. T. Smyke, N. A. Fox, and C. A. Nelson. 2010. Stereotypies in children with a history of early institutional care. *Archives of Pediatrics & Adolescent Medicine* 164(5):406-411.

Bos, K., C. H. Zeanah, N. A. Fox, S. S. Drury, K. A. McLaughlin, and C. A. Nelson. 2011. Psychiatric outcomes in young children with a history of institutionalization. *Harvard Review of Psychiatry* 19(1):15-24.

Browne, K. 2009. *The risk of harm to young children in institutional care.* Fairfield, CT: Save the Children.

Browne, K. D., and S. Chou. 2015. *Mapping the number and characteristics of children in residential care across Europe and Central Asia.* London: Save the Children.

Browne, K., C. Hamilton-Giachritsis, R. Johnson, and M. Ostergren. 2006. Overuse of institutional care for children in Europe. *Child-Care Health and Development* 32(4):502.

Brüggemann, C. 2012. *Roma education in comparative perspective. Findings from the UNDP/World Bank/EC Regional Roma Survey.* Roma Inclusion Working Papers. Bratislava: UNDP.

Cluver, L., M. Orkin, M. E. Boyes, L. Sherr, D. Makasi, and J. Nikelo. 2013. Pathways from parental AIDS to child psychological, educational and sexual risk: Developing an empirically-based interactive theoretical model. *Social Science & Medicine* 87:185-193.

Crenshaw, K. 1989. Demarginalizing the intersection of race and sex: A black feminist critique of antidiscrimination doctrine, feminist theory and antiracist politics. *Univeristy of Chicago Legal Fund* 139.

Csaky, C. 2009. *Keeping children out of harmful institutions: Why we should be investing in family-based care.* Fairfield, CT: Save the Children.

De Laat, J., R. Ali, V. Illieva, C. Sykora, and N. Lepeshko. 2012. *Toward an equal start: Closing the early learning gap for Roma children in Eastern Europe.* Washington, DC: World Bank.

Dowd, A., I. Borisova, and A. Ali. Under review. Realizing capabilities in Ethiopia: Maximizing early childhood investment for impact and equity. *Journal of Human Development and Capabilities.*

Dumcius, R., J. Peeters, N. Hayes, G. Van Landeghem, H. Siarova, L. Peciukoyte, I. Ceneric, and H. Hulpia. 2014. *Study on the effective use of early childhood education and care in preventing early school leaving.* Vilnius, Lithuania: Public Policy and Management Institute.

Dwyer, D. President Obama Offers Legal Status to Millions of Undocumented Immigrants. *ABC News, November 2014.* http://abcnews.go.com/Politics/president-obama-offer-legal-status-millions-undocumented-immigrants/story?id=27063573 (accessed February 8, 2016).

Embleton, L., D. Ayuku, A. Kamanda, L. Atwoli, S. Ayaya, R. Vreeman, W. Nyandiko, P. Gisore, J. Koech, and P. Braitstein. 2014. Models of care for orphaned and separated children and upholding children's rights: Cross-sectional evidence from western Kenya. *BMC International Health and Human Rights* 14(1):1.

Ertem, I. O. 2015. *Developmental Difficulties in Early Childhood: Survey Report.* UNICEF RO CEE/CIS, Geneva.

Ertem I. O., D. G. Dogan, C. G. Gok, S. U. Kizilates, A. Caliskan, G. Atay, N. Vatandas, T. Karaaslan, S. G. Baskan, and D. V. Cicchetti. 2008. A guide for monitoring child development in low-and middle-income countries. *Pediatrics* 121(3):e581-e589.

European Roma Rights Centre. 2011. *Life sentence: Romani children in institutional care.* Budapest, Hungary: Bulgarian Helsinki Committee, Milan Simecka Foundation and Osservazione.

Evans, P. 2013. *Evaluation of implementation of the National Strategy & Action Plan for the reform of the residential childcare system in Moldova 2007–2012.* New York: UNICEF.

Fernald, L. C., P. Kariger, M. Hidrobo, and P. J. Gertler. 2012. Socioeconomic gradients in child development in very young children: Evidence from India, Indonesia, Peru, and Senegal. *Proceedings of the National Academy of Sciences of the United States of America* 109(Suppl 2):17273-17280.

Fleck, G. 2008. *Come closer. Inclusion and exclusion of Roma in present day Romanian society.* Romania: Human Dynamics. Cosima Rughinis.

Fox, N. A., A. N. Almas, K. A. Degnan, C. A. Nelson, and C. H. Zeanah. 2011. The effects of severe psychosocial deprivation and foster care intervention on cognitive development at 8 years of age: Findings from the Bucharest Early Intervention Project. *Journal of Child Psychology and Psychiatry* 52(9):919-928.

Gabal Analysis and Consulting. 2015. Analýza sociálneˇ vyloucˇených lokalit v CˇR [Mapping Analysis of Socially Excluded Localities in the Czech Republic (2015) www.gac.cz/userfiles/File/nase_ prace_vystupy/Analyza_socialne_vyloucenych_lokalit_GAC.pdf (accessed February 8, 2016).

Gordon, I. 2015. There will be fewer child migrants this year, but the crisis isn't over. *Mother Jones* February 13. http://www.motherjones.com/politics/2015/02/unaccompanied-child-migrants-surge-mexico-violence (accessed February 18, 2016).

Gray, C. L., B. W. Pence, J. Ostermann, R. A. Whetten, K. O'Donnell, N. M. Thielman, and K. Whetten. 2015. Prevalence and incidence of traumatic experiences among orphans in institutional and family-based settings in 5 low-and middle-income countries: A longitudinal study. *Global Health: Science and Practice* 3(3):395-404.

Government of FYR Macedonia. 2008. National Strategy for Deinstitutionalization 2008–2018.

Government of FYR Macedonia. 2010. National Strategy for Equalization of the Rights of People with Disabilities in Macedonia 2010–2018.

Hamilton-Giachritsis, C., and K. Browne. 2012. Forgotten children? An update on young children in institutions across Europe. *Early Human Development* 88(12):911-914.

HHS and ED (U.S. Department of Health and Human Services and U.S. Department of Education). 2016. Policy Statement on Inclusion of Children With Disabilities in Early Childhood Programs: September 14, 2015. *Infants & Young Children* 29(1):3-24. doi: 10.1097/iyc.0000000000000054.

Hillis, S., J. Mercy, J. Saul, J. Gleckel, N. Abad, and H. Kress. 2015. THRIVES: A global technical package to prevent violence against children. Atlanta, GA: Centers for Disease Control and Prevention.

Hix-Small, H. 2015. *Early childhood intervention: Global survey results*. Presentation to the Forum on Investing in Young Children Globally. Prague, Czech Republic.

Human Rights Watch. 2015. *US: First step to end family immigration detention*. Human Rights Watch news release, June 24. https://www.hrw.org/news/2015/06/24/us-first-step-end-family-immigration-detention (accessed February 18, 2016).

Humphreys, K. L., M. M. Gleason, S. S. Drury, D. Miron, C. A. Nelson, N. A. Fox, and C. H. Zeanah. 2015. Effects of institutional rearing and foster care on psychopathology at age 12 years in Romania: Follow-up of an open, randomised controlled trial. *Lancet Psychiatry* 2(7):625-634.

International Committee of the Red Cross, International Rescue Commission, Save the Children, UNICEF, United Nations High Commissioner for Refugees, and World Vision. 2004. *Inter-Agency Guiding Principles on Unaccompanied and Separated Children*, January 2004. http://www.refworld.org/docid/4113abc14.html (accessed April 18, 2016).

IOM and NRC (Institute of Medicine and National Research Council). 2000. *From neurons to neighborhoods: The science of early childhood development*. Washington, DC: National Academy Press.

Ivatts, A., K. Cada, L. Felcmanova, D. Greger, and J. Strakova. 2015. *Roma Early Childhood Inclusion+: Special report on Roma inclusion in early childhood education and care*. Czech Republic: Open Society Foundations, UNICEF, and Roma Education Fund.

Klaus, S. 2014. *Straggling behind: Participation of Roma children and employment of Roma staff in early childhood education in Europe*. London, UK: Faculty of Children and Learning, Institute of Education at University of London.

Krishnamurthy, V. 2015. *Monitoring early childhood development in low resource settings using the GMCD*. Presentation to the Forum on Investing in Young Children Globally. Prague, Czech Republic.

The Law on Primary Education. Official Gazette of the Republic of Macedonia No. 51/2007.

Li, X., D. Barnett, X. Fang, X. Lin, G. Zhao, and J. Zhao. 2009. Lifetime incidences of traumatic events and mental health among children affected by HIV/AIDS in rural China. *Journal of Clinical Child & Adolescent Psychology* 38(5):731-744.

Lumos. 2009. Evaluation of situation and needs in child protection at local level. Moldova. (unpublished data).

Malanciuc, I. 2015. *Lumos model for deinstitutionalisation: Improving the lives of marginalised children*. Presentation to the Forum on Investing in Young Children Globally. Prague, Czech Republic.

Matache, M. 2014. *Social ecology of young Romani children: Risk and protective factors for their development: A case study on Romania*. Romania: Editura Publica.

McDermott, J. M., S. Troller-Renfree, R. Vanderwert, C. A. Nelson, C. H. Zeanah, and N. A. Fox. 2013. Psychosocial deprivation, executive functions, and the emergence of socio-emotional behavior problems. *Frontiers in Human Neuroscience* 7:167.

McDonald, C. and K. Negrin. 2010. *No data—no progress: Data collection in countries participating in the decade of Roma Inclusion 2005–2010*. New York: Open Society Foundations.

Merz, E. C., R. B. McCall, and V. Groza. 2013. Parent-reported executive functioning in postinstitutionalized children: A follow-up study. *Journal of Clinical Child & Adolescent Psychology* 42(5):726-733.

Ministry of Labor and Social Policy. 2008. National Strategy for Deinstitutionalization 2008–2018. Skopje: 2014.

Morantz, G., D. Cole, R. Vreeman, S. Ayaya, D. Ayuku, and P. Braitstein. 2013. Child abuse and neglect among orphaned children and youth living in extended families in sub-Saharan Africa: What have we learned from qualitative inquiry? *Vulnerable Children and Youth Studies* 8(4):338-352.

National Center for Farmworker Health. 2012. *Child labor in agriculture*. http://www.ncfh.org/uploads/3/8/6/8/38685499/fs-child_labor.pdf (accessed February 18, 2016).

National ECCD (Early Childhood Care and Development) Impact Evaluation Study 2015, Save the Children Bhutan with the Ministry of Education of Bhutan, http://resourcecentre.savethechildren.se/library/national-eccd-impact-evaluation-study-2015 (accessed February 10, 2016).

Nelson, C. A., C. H. Zeanah, N. A. Fox, P. J. Marshall, A. T. Smyke, and D. Guthrie. 2007. Cognitive recovery in socially deprived young children: The Bucharest Early Intervention Project. *Science* 318(5858):1937-1940.

Nelson, C., N. Fox, and C. Zeanah. 2014. *Romania's abandoned children: Deprivation, brain development, and the struggle for recovery*. Cambridge, MA: Harvard University Press.

Oweini, A. I., and G. Issa. 2015. Evaluating MOCEP's pilot program in Lebanon in Palestinian camps. In *Education applications & developments*, edited by M. Carmo. Lisboa, Portugal: Science Press. Pp. 142-147.

The Parliament of the Republic of Macedonia. 2004. The National Strategy for the Development of Education in the Republic of Macedonia. 2005–2015.

Peeters, J., and N. Sharmahd. 2014. Professional development for ECEC practitioners with responsibilities for children at risk: Which competences and in-service training are needed? *European Early Childhood Education Research Journal* 22(3):412-424.

Peeters, J., and A. Vandekerckhove. 2015. A meeting place for policy-makers and researchers: The Transatlantic Forum on Inclusive Early Years. *International Journal of Early Years Education* 23(3):329-337.

Pilkington, E. 2015a. Migrant family detention under new scrutiny after mother attempts suicide. *The Guardian*, June 6. http://www.theguardian.com/us-news/2015/jun/06/family-detention-centers-renewed-scrutiny-migrant-mother-suicide-attempt (accessed February 8, 2016).

Pilkington, E. 2015b. Soul-destroying: One migrant mother's story of life at Dilley detention center. *The Guardian*, May 22. http://www.theguardian.com/us-news/2015/may/22/immigrant-mothers-dilley-family-detention-center-texas (accessed February 8, 2016).

Pisani, L., I. Borisova, and A. Dowd. 2015. *International development and early learning assessment technical paper.* Fairfield, CT: Save the Children.

Preston, J. 2015. Judge orders release of immigrant children detained by U.S. *The New York Times.* http://www.nytimes.com/2015/07/26/us/detained-immigrant-children-judge-dolly-gee-ruling.html (accessed February 8, 2016).

Raikes, A. 2015. *Measurement birth to age 8.* Presentation to the Forum on Investing in Young Children Globally. Prague, Czech Republic.

Ravnbøl, C. I. 2009. *Intersectional discrimination against children: Discrimination against Romani children and anti-discrimination measures to address child trafficking.* Florence: UNICEF Innocenti Research Centre.

Reza, A., M. J. Breiding, J. Gulaid, J. A. Mercy, C. Blanton, Z. Mthethwa, S. Bamrah, L. L. Dahlberg, and M. Anderson. 2009. Sexual violence and its health consequences for female children in Swaziland: A cluster survey study. *Lancet* 373(9679):1966-1972. doi: 10.1016/S0140-6736(09)60247-6.

Rodríguez, N. S., and N. Rodríguez. 2009. *Health and the Roma community, Analysis of the situation in Europe: Bulgaria, Czech Republic, Greece, Portugal, Romania, Slovakia, Spain.* Madrid: Fundación Secretariado Gitano.

Smyke, A. T., S. F. Koga, D. E. Johnson, N. A. Fox, P. J. Marshall, C. A., Nelson. C. H. Zeanah, and BEIP Core Group. 2007. The caregiving context in institution-reared and family-reared infants and toddlers in Romania. *Journal of Child Psychology and Psychiatry* 48(2):210-218.

Son Hing, L. 2012. Responses to stigmatization: The moderating roles of primary and secondary appraisals. *Du Bois Review* 9:149-168.

St. Petersburg–USA Orphanage Research Team. 2008. The effects of early social-emotional and relationship experience on the development of young orphanage children. *Monographs of the Society for Research in Child Development* 73(3):vii.

Sumner, S. A., A. A. Mercy, J. Saul, N. Motsa-Nzuza, G. Kwesigabo, R. Buluma, L. Marcelin, H. Lina, M. Shawa, M. Moloney-Kitts, T. Kilbane, C. Sommarin, D. Ligiero, K. Brookmeyer, L. Chiang, V. Lea, J. Lee, H. Kress, and S. Hillis. 2015. Prevalence of sexual violence against children and use of social services-seven countries, 2007–2013. *Morbidity and Mortality Weekly Report* 64(21):565-569.

Thera, P., L. Pisani, M. Bamadio, Y. Griffiths, R. Jones, and S. Clarke. 2015. *Measuring child health, cognition and child development: A Malian experience.* Washington, DC: Comparative and International Education Society.

Todres, J. 2011. Mainstreaming children's rights in post-disaster settings. *Emory International Law Review* 25:1233-1261.

Todres, J. 2014. Independent children and the legal construction of childhood. *Southern California Interdisciplinary Law Journal* 23:261-304.

UN (United Nations) General Assembly. 1951. *Convention Relating to the Status of Refugees,* 28 July 1951, United Nations, Treaty Series, vol. 189. http://www.refworld.org/docid/3be01b964.html (accessed April 18, 2016).

UN General Assembly. 2015. *Transforming our world: The 2030 agenda for sustainable development.* New York: UN General Assembly.

UNDP (United Nations Development Programme). 2012. *The situation of Roma in 11 EU member states: Survey results at a glance.* France: European Union Agency for Fundamental Rights.

UNDP-World Bank Roma survey 2011, UNICEF database 2012 for school year 2010/2011, European Union Agency for Fundamental Rights survey 2011.

UNESCO (United Nations Educational, Scientific and Cultural Organization). 2016. *Glossary*. http://www.unesco.org/new/en/social-and-human-sciences/themes/international-migration/glossary/asylum-seeker (accessed April 14, 2016).

UNHCR (United Nations High Commissioner for Refugees). 2014. *UNHCR Global Trends: Forced discplacement in 2014: World at War*. http://unhcr.org/556725e69.html (accessed April 18, 2016).

UNHCR. 2015a. *Global facts and figures for displaced individuals*. Geneva, Switzerland: UNHCR.

UNHCR. 2015b. *UNHCR Refugee Resettlement Trends 2015*. http://www.refworld.org/docid/55aca1864.html (accessed April 18, 2016).

UNHCR. n.d. UNHCR Syria Regional Refugee Response. http://data.unhcr.org/syrian refugees/regional.php (accessed April 18, 2016).

UNICEF (United Nations Children's Fund). 1989. *Convention on the Rights of the Child*. New York: UNICEF.

UNICEF. 2005. Child abandonment in the Republic of Moldova. In *UNICEF and the Government of the Republic of Moldova*, coordinated by I. Malanciuc, D. Ginu, S. Lupan. New York: UNICEF. http://www.unicef.org/moldova/ro/rom_Abandonment_of_young_child.pdf (accessed March 5, 2016).

UNICEF. 2009. *Progress for children: A report card on child protection*. New York: UNICEF.

UNICEF. 2011. *The right of Roma children to education*. Position paper. Paris, France: UNICEF.

UNICEF. 2013. *Children with disabilities*. New York: UNICEF.

UNICEF. 2014. *Inclusive early childhood development and disability: Programme guidance*. New York: UNICEF.

UNICEF. 2015. *Orphans*. http://www.unicef.org/media/media_45279.html (accessed March 23, 2016).

Urban Institute. 2004. *The health and well-being of young children of immigrants*. http://www.urban.org/sites/default/files/alfresco/publication-pdfs/311139-The-Health-and-Well-Being-of-Young-Children-of-Immigrants.PDF (accessed February 18, 2016).

Vandenbroeck, M., and A. Lazzari. 2014. Accessibility of early childhood education and care: A state of affairs. *European Early Childhood Education Research Journal* 22(3):327-335.

Vanderwert, R. E., P. J. Marshall, C. A. Nelson III, C. H. Zeanah, and N. A. Fox. 2010. Timing of intervention affects brain electrical activity in children exposed to severe psychosocial neglect. *PLoS ONE* 5(7):e11415.

Vargas-Baron, E., and J. Schipper. 2012. *Review of policy and planning indicators in early childhood*. Washington, DC: RISE Institute.

Wertlieb, D. 2015. *Special needs, special rights: Investing in children with disabilities through inclusive early childhood development*. Presentation to the Forum on Investing in Young Children Globally. Prague, Czech Republic.

Whetten, K., J. Ostermann, B. W. Pence, R. A. Whetten, L. C. Messer, S. Ariely, K. O'Donnell. A. I. Wasonga, V. Vann, D. Itemba, I. Madan, N. Thielman, and Positive Outcomes for Orphans (POFO) Research Team. 2014. Three-year change in the wellbeing of orphaned and separated children in institutional and family-based care settings in five low-and middle-income countries. *PLoS ONE* 9(8):e104872.

WHO (World Health Organization). 2016. *Global Health Observatory data: Under-five mortality*. Geneva, Switzerland: WHO.

Windsor, J., J. P. Benigno, C. A. Wing, P. J. Carroll, S. F. Koga, C. A. Nelson, N. A. Fox, and C. H. Zeanah. 2011. Effect of foster care on young children's language learning. *Child Development* 82(4):1040-1046.

World Bank. 2015. *Incheon declaration: Education 2030 - towards inclusive and equitable quality education and lifelong learning for all.* Washington, DC: World Bank Group. http://documents.worldbank.org/curated/en/2015/12/25662441/incheon-declaration-education-2030-towards-inclusive-equitable-quality-education-lifelong-learning-all (accessed April 4, 2016).

Yousafzai, T., and M. Rasheed. 2015. *The impact of a pilot integrated early childhood development service on young children and their families: Lessons learned for programme expansion and policy advocacy.* Geneva, Switzerland: UNICEF.

Appendix A

Abbreviations and Acronyms

ACEV	Mother Child Education Foundation
ACF	Albanian Children's Foundation
ASQ	Ages and Stages Questionnaire
ASQ: I	Ages and Stages Questionnaire: Inventory
CDC	U.S. Centers for Disease Control and Prevention
CEE/CIS	Central and Eastern Europe and the Commonwealth of Independent States
ECI	early childhood intervention
GMCD	Guide for Monitoring Child Development
HIV	human immunodeficiency virus
IDELA	International Development and Early Learning Assessment
IQ	intelligence quotient
ISSA	International Step by Step Association
iYCG Forum	Forum on Investing in Young Children Globally
MDG	Millennium Development Goal
NGO	nongovernmental organization

RECI	Roma Early Childhood Inclusion
SEAN	South European Autism Network
THRIVES	Training, Household, Reduce, Improve, Value, Educate, Surveillance
UN CRC	United Nations Convention on the Rights of the Child
UN CRPD	United Nations Convention on the Rights of Persons with Disabilities
UN SDG	United Nations Sustainable Development Goal
UNDP	United Nations Development Programme
UNESCO	United Nations Educational, Scientific and Cultural Organization
UNHCR	United Nations High Commissioner for Refugees
UNICEF	United Nations Children's Fund
VACS	Violence Against Children Surveys
WHO	World Health Organization

Appendix B

Workshop Agenda

Forum on Investing in Young Children Globally (iYCG)
Workshop 6
Reaching and Investing in Children at the Margins

Held in partnership with the Open Society Foundations and the International Step by Step Association (ISSA)
Diplomat Hotel

Prague, Czech Republic
November 3–4, 2015

In September 2015, the Sustainable Development Goals (SDGs) for 2015–2030 were adopted at the United Nations. The global goals reflect the striving for a world that is "just, equitable, and inclusive." They recognize that far too many children are born into and raised in abject poverty. Many children face multiple disadvantages, and all too often live on the margins, excluded—together with their families and caregivers—from full participation in society. These include children with developmental delays and disabilities, refugees, immigrants, migrants, street children, those living in institutions, ethnically and linguistically diverse children, and children from underresourced communities, many of which, like the Roma communities in Europe, face deep discrimination.

An ad hoc planning committee will plan and conduct an interactive public workshop featuring presentations and discussions that highlight the science and economics of investing in children at the margins of society by investing in their health, education, nutrition, and social protection. This workshop, the sixth in the iYCG Forum series, brings to the foreground a scientific perspective on children at the margins. The workshop will include a critical review of the implementation of the Convention on the Rights of the Child as it applies to young children, as well as an exploration of how discrimination and social exclusion affect early development. Subsequent sessions will focus on new information about children living at the margins. The effect of discrimination on young children from underresourced groups will be explored using the example of Roma children in Europe.

The results of the workshop will inform research, policy, and practice in the region as well as globally. The committee will identify specific topics to be addressed, develop the agenda, select and invite speakers and other participants, and moderate the discussions. A summary of the presentations and discussions at the workshop will be prepared by a designated rapporteur in accordance with institutional guidelines. Communications and dissemination products will be drawn from workshop proceedings.

Planning Committee

Liana Ghent, International Step by Step Association (ISSA) (Workshop Co-Chair)
Jody Heymann, University of California, Los Angeles
Gillian Huebner, Lumos Foundation
Tina Hyder, Open Society Foundations
Petra Kacirkova, Lumos Foundation
Sarah Klaus, Open Society Foundations (Workshop Co-Chair)
Vesna Kutlesic, *Eunice Kennedy Shriver* National Institute of Child Health and Human Development
Joan Lombardi, Bernard van Leer Foundation
Ann Masten, University of Minnesota, Minneapolis
Simon Sommer, Jacobs Foundation
Amalia Waxman, Consultant

TUESDAY, NOVEMBER 3
ROOM: PRAHA B, C, AND D
PUBLIC SESSION

8:30–9:00 Introductory Remarks

- **Welcome** (Nives Milinovic, ISSA, and Hirokazu Yoshikawa, Open Society Foundations [OSF], Early Childhood Program Advisory Board)
- **iYCG Overview** (Zulfiqar Bhutta and Ann Masten, iYCG Co-Chairs)
- **Workshop Goals and Objectives** (Sarah Klaus and Liana Ghent, workshop Co-Chairs)

9:00–9:30 Keynote: Young children's rights and the impact of discrimination

Objective: Define global commitments to young children at the margins of society and examine the impact of discrimination on early development in the context of the Convention on the Rights of the Child and the Sustainable

Development Goals. Examine the promises and gaps of these commitments and discuss areas to increase investments in vulnerable young children.

Moderator: Liana Ghent, Executive Director, ISSA
- Share "Poll Everywhere" responses from audience members about expectations of the workshop and challenges and barriers to investing in children at the margins.

Speaker:
- **Jonathan Todres,** Professor of Law, Georgia State University [by pre-recorded video]

9:30–10:45 Session 1: Children living outside of family care
Objective: Develop a new understanding of the developmental impacts on children living in institutions, in foster care, or a nonfamily context. The session will trace a path from global science to prevalence rates in Europe, and impacts and prevention strategies used in the region.

Moderator: Vesna Kutlesic, Director, Office of Global Health, *Eunice Kennedy Shriver* National Institute of Child Health and Human Development

Speakers:
- **Kevin Browne,** Director, Centre for Forensic and Family Psychology, Nottingham University
- **Anne Berens,** Julius B. Richmond Fellow, Harvard University
- **Irina Malanciuc,** Country Director, Lumos Foundation, Moldova

Policy Reaction:
- **Katerina Slesingerova,** Head, Department for Family, Ministry of Labor and Social Affairs, Czech Republic

10:45–11:15 BREAK

11:15–12:30 Session 2: Ethnic and linguistic diversity: The case of young Roma children in Europe
Objective: As the Roma is Europe's largest and most excluded ethnic minority, this session aims to highlight the

context and conditions of young Roma children in Europe. It will consider the risk and protective factors impacting young Roma children, explore new research such as the Roma Early Childhood Initiative (RECI) report for the Czech Republic, and attempt to understand the policy challenges and barriers in Europe to full inclusion of young Roma children.

Moderators:
- **Sarah Klaus,** Director of the Early Childhood Program, Open Society Foundations
- **Iliana Sarafian,** Program Officer, Open Society Foundations

Speakers:
- **Margareta Matache,** Instructor, FXB Center for Health and Human Rights, Harvard University
- **David Greger,** Deputy Director, Institute for Research and Development of Education, Charles University

Policy Reaction:
- **Arthur Ivatts,** Senior Consultant, Open Society Foundations

Research Reaction:
- **Radosveta Dimitrova**, COFAS (create opportunities for collaboration and knowledge sharing) Forte Marie Curie Fellow, Stockholm University, Sweden

12:30–1:30 LUNCH

1:30–2:45 Session 3: Children with developmental delays and disabilities, and atypically developing children

Objective: Explore global efforts to identify and provide services to young children with disabilities and developmental delays and those developing atypically. The session will include a discussion of early childhood interventions available throughout Europe with an emphasis on policy.

Moderator: Andy Shih, Senior Vice President, Scientific Affairs, Autism Speaks

Speakers:

- **Vibha Krishnamurthy,** Founder and Director, Ummeed Child Development Center
- **Donald Wertlieb,** Partnership for Early Childhood Development and Disability Rights (PECDDR)
- **Hollie Hix-Small,** Assistant Professor, Portland State University, and Consultant, Early Childhood Intervention

Policy Reaction Panel:

- **Liri Berisha,** former first lady of Albania, and President, Albanian Children's Foundation
- **Maia Buchukuri,** Social Service Agency (SSA) Head of Social Programs, Division Guardianship-Custody and Social Programs Department, Ministry of Health, Georgia
- **Ariel Com**o, Albanian National Coordinator for South European Autism Network (SEAN)
- **Lidija Dojcinovska,** State Advisor, Office of the Prime Minister, Macedonia
- **Bettina Schwethelm,** Senior Consultant, Young Child Health and Wellbeing, UNICEF Regional Office for Central Eastern Europe and the Commonwealth of Independent States
- **Tatjana Zorcec,** National Coordinator for Autism, Macedonia

2:45–4:00 **Session 4: Children on the move: Migrants, immigrants, and refugees**

Objective: Highlight strategies to reach young migrant children, immigrants, and refugees around the world, with a particular focus on the current refugee crisis in Europe. Speakers will address policies and programs that target displaced children and suggest opportunities to invest in this vulnerable population.

Moderator: Joan Lombardi, Senior Advisor, Bernard van Leer Foundation

Speakers:

- **Eskinder Negash,** Senior Vice President for Global Engagement, U.S. Committee for Refugees and Immigrants

- **Suna Hanoz,** Senior Specialist, Mother Child Education Foundation (ACEV) in Turkey
- **Alison Parker,** Director, U.S. Programs, Human Rights Watch

Research Reaction:

- **Jan Peeters,** Director of Innovations in the Early Years, Research Centre for Early Childhood Education and Care (VBJK), Ghent University

4:00–4:15 BREAK

4:15–5:30 Breakout Sessions: Examples of good practices

Breakout 1: Children living outside of family care
(Belvedere I and II rooms)

- **Lead: Irina Malanciuc,** Country Director, Lumos Foundation, Moldova
- **Perspective: Sevdzihan Ejubova,** Karin Dom, Bulgaria

Breakout 2: Ethnic and linguistic diversity: The case of young Roma children in Europe
(Belvedere III and IV rooms)

- **Lead: Margareta Matache,** Instructor, FXB Center for Health and Human Rights, Harvard University
- **Perspectives: Bozidar Nikolic,** ROMANIPEN, Serbia, and **Miroslav Sklenka,** Step by Step Slovakia

Breakout 3: Children with developmental delays and disabilities, and atypically developing children
(Praha A room)

- **Lead: Donald Wertlieb,** PECDDR
- **Perspective: Mariana Nikolova,** Karin Dom, Bulgaria

Breakout 4: Children on the move: Migrants, immigrants, and refugees
(Praha B, C, and D rooms)

- **Lead: Alison Parker,** Human Rights Watch

5:30–6:15 Bringing it together: Report out and closing discussion

- **Moderator: Amalia Waxman,** Consultant

WEDNESDAY, NOVEMBER 4
ROOM: PRAHA B, C, AND D
PUBLIC SESSION

Half Day Session on Measurement Tools
Objective: Examine efforts to combine child development and quality measurement to support early childhood development (ECD) programs and policies, and provide an overview and discussion of several measurement tools related to child education, nutrition, health, and social protection.

Moderator: Hirokazu Yoshikawa, Courtney Sale Ross University Professor of Globalization and Education, New York University

8:30–9:30 Keynote: Combining child development and quality measurement to support ECD programs and policies

- Measuring Early Learning and Quality Outcomes (MELQO) and WHO Child Indicator Group
  — **Abbie Raikes,** Technical Development Lead, UNICEF

Presentations and discussion about measurement tools

9:30–9:45 ASQ Inventory—**Hollie Hix Small,** Assistant Professor, Portland State University

9:45–10:00 IDELA—**Ivelina Borisova,** Director for Impact and Innovations, Early Childhood Development, Save the Children

10:00–10:15 Guide for Monitoring Child Development (GMCD)—**Vibha Krishnamurthy,** Ummeed Child Development Center

10:15–10:30 Violence Against Children Surveys (VACS)—**Ruth Perou,** CDC [by pre-recorded video]

10:30–11:00 BREAK

11:00–11:15 **Policy Reaction: Emily Vargas-Barón,** Director, RISE Institute

11:15–11:45 **Moderated Discussion,** Hiro Yoshikawa, New York University

11:45–12:00 Closing Remarks (Sarah Klaus and Liana Ghent, workshop Co-Chairs)

12:00 Adjourn

Appendix C

Biographical Sketches of Workshop Speakers

Anne Berens, M.Sc., M.A., is a Richmond Fellow at the Center on the Developing Child at Harvard University and researcher at the Laboratories of Cognitive Neuroscience at Children's Hospital Boston. Her research focuses on the measurement and neurodevelopmental effects of early childhood psychosocial adversity in low-income countries. She has particular interest in the effects of early care environments on developmental outcomes, and in the needs of children lacking access to safe family settings.

Liri Berisha was graduated by the Faculty of Medicine, University of Tirana, and has worked as a pediatrician for 30 years. As president of the Albanian Children's Foundation and in support of its mission she is focused on creating opportunities for the education of marginalized children, improving care and development in early childhood, protecting the rights of children, the healthy growing of children with special physical and social needs, and improving the lives of children suffering from thalassemia, contributing to sustainable solutions to their problems. Mrs. Berisha has made possible the increasing public and professional awareness of autism in Albania. She has introduced programs and international standardized instruments for screening, diagnosing, providing quality treatment services, and increasing professional capacities for children with autism spectrum disorder, and she has developed academic editions to strengthen inclusive programs and multiple efforts at the international level coordinating and establishing a sustainable national model to provide professional services. Her engagement in many national and international activities, reducing infant mortality in the country, and initiating the establishment of several international networks for improving the lives of children is considered by worldwide dignitaries as a global role model, bestowing her with such prestigious awards as the Order of Mother Teresa by the President of the Republic of Albania, the Second Annual Bob and Suzanne Wright Global Autism Achievement Award, and Honorary President and Local Ambassador of UNICEF.

Zulfiqar Bhutta, MBBS, FRCPCH, FAAP, Ph.D., is the Robert Harding Inaugural Chair in Global Child Health at The Hospital for Sick Children (SickKids), Toronto, the codirector of the SickKids Centre for Global Child Health, and Founding Director of the Centre of Excellence in Women and Child Health, at the Aga Khan University, unique joint appointments. He also holds adjunct professorships at the Schools of Public Health at Johns Hopkins University (Baltimore), Tufts University (Boston), the University of Alberta, and the London School of Hygiene & Tropical Medicine. He is a designated Distinguished National Professor of the Government of Pakistan and was the founding chairman of the National Research Ethics Committee of the Government of Pakistan from 2002–2014. Dr. Bhutta's research interests include newborn and child survival, maternal and child undernutrition, and micronutrient deficiencies. Dr. Bhutta is one of the seven-member Independent Expert Review Group (iERG) established by the United Nations Secretary General in September 2011 for monitoring global progress in maternal and child health Millennium Development Goals (MDGs). He represents the global academic and research organizations on the Global Alliance for Vaccines and Immunizations (GAVI) Board, is the cochair of the Maternal and Child Health oversight committee of World Health Organization Regional Office for the Eastern Mediterranean (WHO EMRO) as well as the Global Countdown for 2015 Steering Group. He has served as a member of the Global Advisory Committee for Health Research for the WHO, the Board of Child & Health and Nutrition Initiative of the Global Forum for Health Research, and was a founding board member of the Global Partnership for Maternal, Newborn and Child Health (PMNCH). He serves on several international editorial boards. Dr. Bhutta is currently a member of the WHO Strategic Advisory Committee for Vaccines (SAGE), the Expert Advisory Group for Vaccine Research, the Advisory Committee for Health Research of WHO EMRO, and a cochair of its apex Regional Committee for Maternal and Child Health. He has won several awards, including the Aga Khan University Awards for Research (2005) Distinguished Faculty (2012), and the WHO Ihsan Dogramaci Family Health Award (2014). Professor Bhutta received his Ph.D. from the Karolinska Institute, Sweden, and is a Fellow of the Royal College of Pediatrics & Child Health, American Academy of Pediatrics, and the Pakistan Academy of Sciences.

Ivelina Borisova, Ph.D., Director for Impact and Innovations, Early Childhood Development at Save the Children, brings extensive expertise in international early childhood programs and policy. Dr. Borisova obtained her doctoral degree in Human Development and Psychology from Harvard University and prior to joining Save the Children, worked as an international consultant with numerous development agencies, including World Education and the International Rescue Committee. Dr. Borisova works on developing, implementing, and evaluating early childhood programs and policies around the world and provides strategic and technical guidance to a diverse portfolio of early childhood development initiatives across Asia, Africa, the Middle East, and Eastern/Central Europe, spanning the full continuum of early childhood (pregnancy to 8 years). At Save the Children, she has strengthened the focus and application of evidence-based programming and promoted a focus on equity and quality in early childhood services. Most recently, Dr. Borisova led the development and validation of the International Development and Early Learning Assessment (IDELA), which is quickly gaining momentum as a global instrument on early learning. Dr. Borisova has published numerous articles and reports, and has presented extensively at conferences, meetings, and workshops (academic and nonacademic) globally.

Kevin Browne, B.Sc. (Hons), M.Sc., Ph.D., M.Ed., C.Psychol., FSB, is Director of the Centre for Forensic and Family Psychology and holds the Chair of Forensic Psychology and Child Health at the University of Nottingham Medical School. He is Consultant to the European Commission, UNICEF, and the World Health Organization on children in adversity and children in conflict with the law, following 12 years as an Executive Councilor of the International Society for the Prevention of Child Abuse and Neglect. He has worked in more than 50 countries to improve the care and protection of children. With the aid of a European Union Daphne grant, he co-developed a model for deinstitutionalizing and transforming children's services in Europe, which has been used by UNICEF (Better Care Network), Hope & Homes, and Lumos. In 2009, his work on risk of harm to young children was influential in bringing about United Nations guidelines that *no* child less than 3 should be placed in residential care without a parent. In 2013, with Open Society Foundations support, he again mapped the number of children in care across Europe and Central Asia together with UNICEF to compare changes from 2003.

Maia Buchukuri, M.D., is currently Head of the Social Programs Division in the Ministry of Labor, Health, and Social Affairs, Social Service Agency in Georgia. Since its founding, Dr. Buchukuri has been the coordinator of the governmental program of Early Intervention, and is a member of the Early Intervention Coalition. Dr. Buchukuri manages other state social programs, including small group homes, child rehabilitation, day care centers, community organizations, and provision of supporting equipment (such as wheelchairs and prosthetic-orthopedic equipment, and hearing devices and cochlear implants).

Ariel Como, M.D., is an Associate Professor of Psychiatry at the Tirana Medical University, is currently clinical Head of Psychiatry Division, Department of Neuroscience, Tirana University Hospital Center "Mother Tereza." Since November 2014 he has been Deputy Dean for Continuing Medical Education at the Faculty of Medicine, Tirana Medical University; a member of the Directors' Council of postgraduate schools in Neurosciences (including General Psychiatry and Child and Adolescent Psychiatry); a member of the National Steering Committee on Reforming the Mental Health Sector, and a member of working group on developing intersectorial strategy on Child and Adolescent Mental Health. During 2008–2014 he served as General Deputy Director of the University Hospital Center. Since 2010 he has been National Coordinator at the South East European Autism Network, and Scientific Director of the Tirana Regional Center on Autism. Dr. Como received his M.D. in 1994 and postgraduate residency in Psychiatry in 1999 at the Tirana Faculty of Medicine; specialization course in Child Neuropsychiatry at the University of Pavia, Italy; and his doctoral degree on trans-generational transmission of trauma at the Tirana University. He served as Consultant for the Albanian Rehabilitation Center on Trauma and Torture, International Organization of Migration, and other nongovernmental actors or programs in different periods. From 2011 to 2016 he has been a postdoc fellow at the University of California, Berkeley, on the research training socio-economics of mental health delivery in southeastern Europe at the Nicholas C. Petris Center.

Radosveta Dimitrova, Ph.D., received her Ph.D. in Developmental Psychology (Trieste University, Italy; awarded 2009 Best Doctoral Thesis, Italian Psychological Association) and Ph.D. in Cross-Cultural Psychology (Tilburg University, the Netherlands, received 2012 Dissertation Award of the Society for Research in Child Development). She worked at the Brent Centre for Young People, London (United Kingdom) and Brown University (United States) and has ongoing collaborations in Africa, Asia, Europe, and the United States. Her publication record includes 55 peer-reviewed scholarly publications and more than 90 presentations and talks at international conferences. Her research interests include migration, positive youth development, marginalized and disadvantaged children and youth, and ethnic minority communities (Roma). She is an Associate Editor of the American Psychological Association's *International Psychology Bulletin*, an ad hoc reviewer of 23 scholarly journals in psychological and related fields, and editor of a book on immigrant families around the globe. She is the past president of the Early Researchers Union of the European Association of Developmental Psychology and current representative of the Early Career Council at the Society for Research in Child Development, the Society for the Study of Human Development, European Association for Research on Adolescence, the Society for Research on Adolescence's Study Group Committee, Society for the Study of Emerging Adulthood Early Career Committee, and Advisory Board of the Global Network for Human Development.

Lidija Dojcinovska, M.A., has a bachelor's degree in special education and rehabilitation and a master's degree in social policy with focus on inclusive education. Since 2000, she has been active in the disability sector in international and national organizations, working on various development projects. Ms. Dojcinovska is co-founder and president of the association Open the Windows, which promotes and provides assistive technology for people with disabilities in Macedonia. Also, she is coauthor of several publications in the field of assistive technology. From 2010 to 2015 she was actively involved in promoting inclusion of children with disabilities, working as a special educator in the mainstream schools in Skopje. As of May 2015, Dr. Dojcinovska is a state advisor in the Prime Minister's office of the Republic of Macedonia.

Liana Ghent joined the International Step by Step Association (ISSA) as Executive Director in September 2006. She is responsible for the day-to-day management and strategic development of the association, which brings together more than 65 organizations from close to 40 countries, primarily from Europe and Central Asia. ISSA's members are united around the shared mission to ensure equal access to quality care and education for all young children from birth to 10 years old. This mission is implemented through three main pillars of action: equal access for all children, promoting high-quality and professionalism in early years services, and empowering parents and communities to be part of children's development and learning. Ms. Ghent has more than 20 years of international experience in developing and leading programs in the nonprofit sector, primarily in the area of higher education and early childhood development. Her leadership experience includes serving as Regional Director and later as President of the Civic Education Project, a nonprofit organization engaged in higher education initiatives in Central and Eastern Europe and the former Soviet Union, during times of intense reforms after the fall of communism. Before joining ISSA, she also worked with the Higher Education Support Program of the Open Society Foundations. She currently serves as a member of the Board of Directors of the Consultative Group on Early Childhood Care and Development.

David Greger, Ph.D., is director of the Institute for Research and Development of Education at Faculty of Education, Charles University, in Prague. He works mainly in the field of comparative education, educational policy, sociology of education, and quantitative methodology. He teaches quantitative research methods and sociology of education for doctoral students and classes on equity in education, educational policy, and quantitative research methods for master's students. His recent work is focused on issues of equity and quality in education, positive discrimination measures for at-risk students, and other policy interventions that may reduce the achievement gaps. Dr. Greger has been involved in many national and international projects and served as an advisor for the European Commission, OECD, Ministry of Education of the Czech Republic, and for several nongovernmental organizations. He currently leads a large longitudinal study in the Czech Republic (CLoSE [Czech Longitudinal Study in Education]) financed by the National Science Foundation of the Czech Republic.

Suna Hanoz, M.A., is currently working as the International Relations Senior Specialist at Mother Child Education Foundation (ACEV). She manages the transfer and implementation of ACEV's educational programs through partnerships with local organizations in numerous countries in Europe, the Middle East, and Central America. Her work focuses on both designing and supervising early intervention projects for children and families implemented in the field. She has authored the Preschool Education Program and the Mother Support Program, along with her colleagues at ACEV. Before ACEV, she taught children at the early childhood level and took part in research studies. Ms. Hanoz is a Fulbright Scholar, received her M.A. degree in Early Childhood Education from Teachers College, Columbia University, and holds a B.A. degree in Early Childhood Education and Psychological Guidance and Counselling from Bogazici University.

Hollie Hix-Small, Ph.D., is an assistant professor and program coordinator for the Early Intervention, Early Childhood Special Education graduate program at Portland State University. Dr. Hix-Small trains master's-level licensure students through a Web-based platform, conducts research, and contributes to the field through international trainings and technical support. Dr. Hix-Small was formerly with Open Society Foundations in London, England, where she managed the organization's early childhood intervention portfolio in Central and Eastern Europe and Eurasia from 2011 to 2014. During her tenure with Open Society Foundations, she facilitated the development of early childhood intervention system building and service provision in several countries. Dr. Hix-Small has worked as an academic in Canada and the United States, served as a home visitor and early childhood special education classroom teacher, worked as an institutional care provider for children ages 0–6, and has been employed as a research analyst on numerous federally funded grants. Dr. Hix-Small's expertise lies in supporting very young children, birth to age 5 and their families, experiencing developmental or social emotional difficulties and research and program evaluation. In 2007 she received her Ph.D. in Early Intervention, Special Education from the University of Oregon. Dr. Hix-Small has trained and consulted on early childhood development and intervention in more than 15 countries.

Arthur Ivatts, M.A., worked initially as a teacher and youth leader. Following a higher degree in anthropology, which focused on the Gypsies/Roma in England, he became involved with the early efforts to secure education for Roma/Gypsy and traveler children. After some years working within the voluntary nongovernmental organization sector concerned with Gypsies/Roma and travelers, he joined Her Majesty's Inspectors of Schools (HMI) in England in 1975 and soon became the HMI with national responsible for the education of Gypsy/Roma and traveler children. He held this post until 2003 when he decided to do consultancy work for government departments and intergovernmental organizations. In 2004, he was awarded an Order of the British Empire by the Queen for his services to education. Mr. Ivatts has been involved in Roma/Gypsy related projects in Albania, Bulgaria, Croatia, Czech Republic, Hungary, Kosovo, Romania, Slovakia, and Sweden. In 2003–2004 he worked with a small research team on a report for the European Commission in relation to Roma and European Union enlargement, *The Situation of Roma in an Enlarged European Union* (EU, November 2004).

Sarah Klaus, M.A., Director of the Open Society Foundations (OSF) Early Childhood Program (ECP), leads a team of specialists who develop and implement the Foundations' global early childhood portfolio. The program improves services and policies that affect young children, particularly minority and marginalized groups, and builds capacity of early childhood professionals. Since 2006, Ms. Klaus has expanded OSF's ECP's original focus in Central Eastern Europe and Eurasia to include Africa, Asia, Latin America, and the Middle East. In 1994, Ms. Klaus helped launch Step by Step, the Foundations' flagship early childhood program, and in 1999, the International Step by Step Association, a network established to support early childhood professionals in Central Eastern Europe and Eurasia. She served as the association's executive director from its inception to 2006. Ms. Klaus holds an M.A. in developmental psychology from Columbia University Teachers College and a B.A. in Russian Studies from Brown University. She is currently pursuing a doctorate in education at the Institute of Education in London.

Vibha Krishnamurthy, M.D., has trained in developmental pediatrics at Children's Hospital, Boston. She founded Ummeed Child Development Center in 2001, a not-for-profit center for children with disability in Mumbai, India. She has 15 years of experience in India as a developmental pediatrician, and has led the team at Ummeed in its delivery of direct services, training, advocacy, and research in the field of child development and disability. She serves on expert committees related to early childhood development and disability for the World Health Organization and government of India. Dr. Krishnamurthy has served on the editorial board of the *Journal of Developmental Behavioral Pediatrics* since 2011. She is currently co-investigator on a project to develop an international tool for monitoring child development, funded by the National Institutes of Health.

Vesna Kutlesic, Ph.D., is the Director of the Office of Global Health at the *Eunice Kennedy Shriver* National Institute of Child Health and Human Development (NICHD). Dr. Kutlesic is also an adjunct faculty member at the Center for Global Health in the School of Public Health at George Washington University. She has served on the Executive Board of the Society for Child and Family Policy and Practice within the American Psychological Association. Previously, Dr. Kutlesic was hired as a Special Assistant to the National Institutes of Health (NIH) Director after completing a mid-career, health science policy fellowship through the American Association for the Advancement of the Sciences. While a Special Assistant in the NIH Director's Office for 4 years, she earned the NIH Director's Award in 2008 for her work on the Revitalizing Peer Review initiative, and worked on research, training, and policy initiatives related to biomedical research, global health, child health, behavioral/social science issues, and interdisciplinary research, among others. Prior to her work at NIH, she was a Fulbright Visiting Professor in the Psychology Department at the University of Belgrade in Serbia, while based in the Psychiatry Department at Case Western Reserve University in Cleveland, Ohio. She has also worked as a senior international consultant for UNICEF on developing children's health and behavioral services in Eastern Europe.

Joan Lombardi, Ph.D., is an international expert on child development and social policy. She currently serves as Senior Advisor to the Buffett Early Childhood Fund on national initiatives and to the Bernard van Leer Foundation on global child development strategies. She also directs Early Opportunities, LLC, focusing on innovation, policy, and philanthropy. Over the past 40 years, Dr. Lombardi has made significant contributions in the areas of child and family policy as an innovative leader and policy advisor to national and international organizations and foundations and as a public servant. She served in the U.S. Department of Health and Human Services as the first Deputy Assistant Secretary for Early Childhood Development (2009–2011) in the Obama administration, and as the Deputy Assistant Secretary for Policy and External Affairs in the Administration for Children and Families, and the first Commissioner of the Child Care Bureau among other positions (1993–1998) during the Clinton administration. Outside of public service, she served as the founding chair of the Birth to Five Policy Alliance (now the Alliance for Early Success) and as the founder of Global Leaders for Young Children. She currently serves on the Board of Trustees for Save the Children and the Board of Directors for the Collaborative for Academic, Social and Emotional Learning.

Irina Malanciuc, Ph.D., has been working as Country Director of Lumos Moldova since 2009, ensuring and coordinating the implementation of Lumos' program in regard to deinstitutionalization, inclusive education, prevention of under-5 mortality, and quality assurance of social services. Dr. Malanciuc started her activity as a pediatrician, working with children at the community level, including children from vulnerable families. She held different positions within the district level, the Institute of Mother and Child Health Care, the Ministry of Health, and UNICEF Moldova. She was involved in national and international projects regarding child protection and the residential child care system, and she coordinated the evaluations of all residential institutions from Moldova (during 1998–1999, 2006–2007, and 2013). The results of these evaluations served as a basis for the reform of the residential child care system. Dr. Malanciuc was also involved, as an UNICEF international expert, in the evaluation of the residential child care system of several post-Soviet countries, and supported the authorities to develop plans for reforming the child care system. Lumos cooperates with the Moldovan government to change the child protection system and ensure the child's right to family, for the benefit of all marginalized children.

Ann Masten, Ph.D., LP, is Regents Professor, Irving B. Harris Professor of Child Development and Distinguished McKnight University Professor in the Institute of Child Development at the University of Minnesota. She completed her doctoral training at the University of Minnesota in clinical psychology and her internship at the University of California, Los Angeles. In 1986, she joined the faculty in the Institute of Child Development at the University of Minnesota, serving as chair of the department from 1999 to 2005. Dr. Masten's research focuses on understanding processes that promote competence and prevent problems in human development, with a focus on adaptive processes and pathways, developmental tasks and cascades, and resilience in the context of high cumulative risk, adversity, and trauma. She directs the Project Competence studies of risk and resilience, including studies of normative populations and high-risk young people exposed to war, natural disasters, poverty, homelessness, and migration. The ultimate objective of her research is to inform sciences, practices, and policies that aim to promote positive development and a better future for children and families whose lives are threatened by adversity. Dr. Masten currently serves on the Board on Children, Youth, and Families (BCYF) and the U.S. National Committee of Psychology for the National Academies of Sciences, Engineering, and Medicine. She formerly served on the BCYF Committee on the Impact of Mobility and Change on the Lives of Young Children, Schools, and Neighborhoods and planning committee on Investing in Young Children Globally. She also has served as President of the Society for Research in Child Development and President of Division 7 (Developmental) of the American Psychological Association (APA). She is a 2014 recipient of the Urie Bronfenbrenner Award for Lifetime Contributions to Developmental Psychology in the Service of Science and Society from APA. Dr. Masten has published and presented extensively on the themes of risk and resilience in human development. Her book, *Ordinary Magic: Resilience in Children*, was published by Guilford Press, and she is teaching a free MOOC (mass open online course) on the same theme beginning in September 2014 on Coursera.

Margareta (Magda) Matache, Ph.D., is a Roma rights activist from Romania. In 2012, she was awarded a Hauser Post-Doctoral Fellowship at the FXB Center for Health and Human Rights at Harvard University. For more than a decade, Dr. Matache has been a powerful voice of the Roma in various grassroots, national, and international contexts. Her views on the Roma plight have been captured and conveyed throughout the world by credible sources, such as *The New York Times*, *The Time*, *Financial Time*, BBC, *EuroNews*, *Le Monde*, and *Le Figaro*, as well as by national media in Romania. From 2005 to 2012, Dr. Matache was the Executive Director of Romani CRISS, a leading Roma nongovernmental organization that defends and promotes the rights of Roma. Their advocacy and litigation efforts have also contributed to the approval of the domestic School Desegregation Bill. She completed her doctoral research work in early childhood development of Romani children at the Faculty of Political Sciences, University of Bucharest, and holds a master's degree in European Social Policies. Her publications and research have ranged over the rights and agency of Romani children and adolescents, early childhood development, Romani women, anti-Roma violence, and segregation in education.

Eskinder Negash is a recognized senior executive leader and brings more than 35 years of proven not-for-profit management experience working on behalf of refugees and immigrants, and managing nonprofit social service agencies. Mr. Negash served as Director of the Office of Refugee Resettlement (ORR), the largest government-funded refugee resettlement organization in the world, within the Administration of Children and Families at the U.S. Department of Health and Human Services from 2009 to 2015. With a budget of more than $1.5 billion, the Office of Refugee Resettlement plays a critical role in providing essential services to a wide range of vulnerable people. Under his leadership, ORR has served more than 400,000 refugees; 150,000 asylees; 125,000 Cuban and Haitian entrants; nearly 21,000 Iraqi and Afghan Special Immigrant Visa holders; 3,200 victims of trafficking; and 116,000 unaccompanied children. Prior to his appointment by the Obama administration, he served as the vice president and chief operating officer of the U.S. Committee for Refugees and Immigrants (USCRI), a nongovernmental, not-for-profit international organization. Before joining USCRI, Mr. Negash served as vice president and chief administrative officer of the International Institute of Los Angeles for 15 years. In 2009, Mr. Negash received an Outstanding American by Choice award from the U.S. Department of Homeland Security U.S. Citizenship and Immigration Services, which recognizes naturalized U.S. citizens who have made significant contributions to both their community and their adopted country. In 2010, the International Rescue Committee (IRC) honored Mr. Negash as 1 of 10 distinguished men and women whose stories of hope and transformation epitomize the refugee journey.

Alison Parker, J.D., director of Human Rights Watch's (HRW's) U.S. Program, guides HRW's work on national security, immigration, and criminal justice in the United States. From 2001 to 2002, she served as a Sandler fellow and the organization's director of refugee policy, in both positions documenting and advocating against violations of the rights of refugees around the world. Ms. Parker has conducted human rights investigations in refugee settings in Africa and Central Asia, as well as in prisons, jails, immigration detention centers, and immigrant communities throughout the United States. She has conducted extensive advocacy before the governments of the United States and Europe; has testified before state legislatures and the U.S. Congress; and is a frequent voice in the media. Ms. Parker has edited and authored numerous HRW reports, including a landmark examination of the sentencing of children to life without the possibility of parole, which was subsequently cited in two U.S. Supreme Court decisions limiting the practice. A graduate of the University of California, Berkeley, and Oxford University, Ms. Parker holds a master's degree from Columbia University's School of International and Public Affairs and a J.D. from Columbia University Law School. Prior to joining HRW, she worked with the United Nations High Commissioner for Refugees, the Jesuit Refugee Service, and engaged in sovereign litigation as an attorney at Cleary Gottlieb Steen and Hamilton in New York.

Jan Peeters, Ph.D., was senior researcher in two research projects commissioned by the European Commission DG E&C (Competences Requirements in Early Childhood Education and Care [ECEC], 2011, and The Role of ECEC in Preventing Early School Leaving, 2014) and he was the promoter of a systematic review for Eurofound on ECEC: Working Conditions, Training and Quality of Services, a Systematic Review (2015). He worked within the IMPRES/UNICEF project that aimed to increase the accessibility of preschool in Serbia. Dr. Peeters and two colleagues from VBJK Innovation in the Early Years, together with the Migration Policy Institute (United States), are responsible for the organization of the Transatlantic Forum on Inclusive Early Years (TFIEY), seven high-level meetings for policy makers and researchers on the importance of quality ECEC for vulnerable groups (2013–2016). He is a member of the United Nations Educational, Scientific and Cultural Organization (UNESCO) International Advisory Group on the Survey of Teachers in Pre-Primary Education (STEPP). He is an elected board member of the International Step by Step Association and the co-founder of the Diversity in Early Childhood Education and Training (DECET) network on working around diversity and inclusion in ECEC.

Ruth Perou, Ph.D., is the Child Development Studies Team Leader at the U.S. Centers for Disease Control and Prevention (CDC), National Center on Birth Defects and Developmental Disabilities (NCBDDD). Dr. Perou is working on implementing CDC's public health agendas on attention-deficit/hyperactivity disorder (ADHD) and Tourette's syndrome and related comorbidities. She is the Project Director of Legacy for Children, CDC's national program to promote optimal child development outcomes in low-income families. Additionally, she is working on the CDC initiative on developmental health, an effort to promote child health and well-being by recognizing the importance of early identification and early intervention for children with or at-risk for developmental delays, developmental disabilities, and childhood disorders. Dr. Perou received her Ph.D.

in Applied Developmental Psychology from the University of Miami in Coral Gables, Florida.

Abbie Raikes, Ph.D., is a developmental psychologist addressing global measurement in early childhood as the technical lead for the Measuring Early Learning Quality and Outcomes project based at UNICEF. Prior to joining UNICEF, Dr. Raikes was a program specialist at the United Nations Educational, Scientific and Cultural Organization (UNESCO) Headquarters in Paris. She also spent several years working on early learning, strategy development, and measurement for The Bill & Melinda Gates Foundation in Seattle, Washington. Dr. Raikes's background also includes training in public health and experience working in the United States Senate on policy.

Bettina Schwethelm, Ph.D., is a Senior Consultant on Young Child Health and Wellbeing at the UNICEF Regional Office for Central, Eastern Europe and the Commonwealth of Independent States (CEE/CIS). She focuses on strengthening the linkages between the areas of health, early child development, and child protection. In her assignment, she supports UNICEF Country Offices and partners on the reform of home visiting services to improve parenting capacities during the critical early years. She supports UNICEF activities for early identification and intervention for children with or at risk of developmental difficulties. She was recently involved in a mapping of services for young children with disabilities or developmental difficulties in CEE/CIS. With a doctorate in developmental psychology and master's degree in International Public Health, she has managed maternal and child health communicable and noncommunicable disease programs in the nongovernmental organization sector for more than 20 years. She has conducted research and published on augmentative communication for nonverbal children and learning disabilities. She is the co-author of a training package for health workers on child-friendly hospital procedures based on child rights, health, and development. She has also co-written two training modules for home visitors on young children with developmental difficulties.

Andy Shih, Ph.D., is Senior Vice President of Scientific Affairs at Autism Speaks. He works closely with members of Autism Speaks' Board, Scientific Advisory Committee, senior staff, and volunteer leadership to develop and implement the organization's research program. He oversees the etiology portfolio, which includes genetics, environmental sciences, and epidemiology, as well as the Innovative Technology for Autism program, which supports the research and development of novel assistive technologies. Dr. Shih also leads Autism Speaks' international scientific development efforts, including the Global Autism Public Health Initiative, an international advocacy effort currently active in more than 45 countries around the world that integrates awareness, research, and service development. His team serves as facilitators and technical advisors to community stakeholders, including government ministries, professional societies, and advocacy organizations. Dr. Shih joined the National Alliance for Autism Research (NAAR) in 2002, an autism science organization that merged with Autism Speaks in 2006. Prior to joining NAAR, he served as an industry consultant and was a member of the faculty at Yeshiva University and New York University Medical Center. Dr. Shih's research background includes published studies in gene identification and characterization, virus–cell interaction, and cell-cycle regulation. He earned his Ph.D. in cellular and molecular biology from New York University Medical Center.

Katerina Slesingerova has been the Director of the Department for the Protection of Children's Rights since June 2015. She graduated from the Law Faculty of Charles University and worked at the Institute for Criminology and Social Prevention, where she participated in the research of juvenile delinquency and the possibilities of its prevention, and researched domestic violence and its impact on children. She has been working more than 15 years in the field of foster care and children living out of their families. She has experience with supporting foster families, counseling, programs for children in institutional care, and research of the needs of young people leaving institutional care. She is actively seeking to change the system of care for vulnerable children in the Czech Republic. She participated in the preparation of the nongovernmental organization report on the United Nations Children's Rights Convention, and presented it at the Committee on the Rights of the Child meeting in 2011. In 2012–2014, she worked at the Ministry of Labour and Social Affairs.

Jonathan Todres, J.D., is Professor of Law at Georgia State University College of Law. His research focuses on children's rights and child well-being, with a particular emphasis on vulnerable populations. Dr. Todres's primary research areas include child trafficking, domestic implementation of children's rights law, economic and social rights issues, and legal and cultural constructs of childhood. Dr. Todres has authored numerous publications on a range of children's rights issues. He also serves as a regular advisor to nongovernmental organizations working on policy initiatives to address children's rights violations. Dr. Todres lectures frequently on children's rights and has presented testimony before the United Nations Committee on the Rights of the Child and at congressional briefings in the U.S. House of Representatives and U.S. Senate on child trafficking and other children's rights issues. Since 2012, Dr. Todres has served on three committees of the National Academies of Sciences, Engineering, and Medicine—two on bullying and one on sex trafficking of minors in the United States. He is a Fellow of the American Bar Foundation. Dr. Todres received his B.A. (International Development) from Clark University and his J.D. from Columbia Law School.

Emily Vargas-Baron, Ph.D., directs The RISE Institute, a global authority on policy development and research in early childhood development (ECD) and early childhood intervention (ECI). Dr. Vargas-Baron also conducts advisory services and research on ECD and ECI policy planning, implementation, and outcomes, serving in more than 25 nations since 2001. From 1994 to 2001, Dr. Vargas-Baron was a Deputy Assistant Administrator for the U.S. Agency for International Development, leading activities in 80 nations for education, telecommunications, and international training. Previously, Dr. Vargas-Baron led an ECD and ECI institute and conducted field research in Austin, Texas; served as an Education Advisor for the Ford Foundation in the Andean Region of Latin America; and was an Education Specialist in the United Nations Educational, Scientific and Cultural Organization focusing on educational planning. Dr. Vargas-Baron has also taught in four universities and authored many books and other publications on ECD, ECI, and educational development. Dr. Vargas-Baron has a Ph.D. in Cognitive Anthropology from Stanford University, with a specialization in international educational planning.

Amalia Waxman, M.A., is an expert in strategy and policy planning, advocacy, private–public partnerships, communications, multistakeholder relations, corporate social responsibility (CSR), international health policy, public affairs, issue and crisis management, and resource development. She is an experienced driver and manager of complex challenging innovative processes and campaigns. Ms. Waxman is also an effective intresectorial negotiator and mediator. She has unique professional experience in private, public, United Nations, and not-for-profit sectors. Some of her noteworthy achievements include leading the development of the World Health Organization's (WHO's) Global Strategy on Diet, Physical Activity and Health, a pivotal global policy in the area of prevention of chronic diseases; adopted by most WHO member states. Ms. Waxman established, branded, and managed a food labeling system—a complex cross-industry CSR initiative. She also developed a national policy on prevention of chronic diseases adopted by the government of Israel.

Donald Wertlieb, Ph.D., is an applied developmental scientist specializing in pediatric psychology, president of the Partnership for Early

Childhood Development and Disability Rights (PECDDR), and professor emeritus at Eliot-Pearson Department of Child Development at Tufts University. He currently coordinates the Early Childhood Development Task Force for the Global Partnership on Children with Disabilities providing access to an international network of policy, program, and research advocates for inclusive early childhood development. He has served as senior consultant since 1998 at the Educational Resource Center for Children with Disabilities in Dnepropetrovsk, Ukraine, providing professional development for Ukrainian colleagues' pioneering efforts in community-based services for children with disabilities and their families. He served as a Fulbright Senior Specialist in Mykolayev, Ukraine. He is a member of the Society for Behavioral and Developmental Pediatrics and the International Society for Early Intervention, and has served as president of both the Society for Pediatric Psychology and the American Orthopsychiatric Association.

Hiro Yoshikawa, Ph.D., is the Courtney Sale Ross University Professor of Globalization and Education at New York University's Steinhardt School of Culture, Education and Human Development. He is also the co-chair of the United Nations Sustainable Development Solutions Network (SDSN) Workgroup on Early Childhood Development, Education, and the Transition to Work, and serves on the Network's Leadership Council. He is a community and developmental psychologist who studies the effects of public policies and programs related to immigration, early childhood, and poverty reduction on children's development. He conducts research in the United States and in low- and middle-income countries, including studies on early childhood development and policy in Cambodia, Chile, Colombia, and other countries. His recent books include *Immigrants Raising Citizens: Undocumented Parents and Their Young Children* (2011, Russell Sage). He has served on the Board on Children, Youth, and Families of the National Academies of Sciences, Engineering, and Medicine; the Early Childhood Advisory Committee of the Inter-American Development Bank; and the U.S. Department of Health and Human Services Advisory Committee on Head Start Research and Evaluation for the Clinton and Obama administrations. In 2011 he was nominated by President Obama and confirmed by the Senate as a member of the U.S. National Board for Education Sciences. In 2013 he was elected to the National Academy of Education. He obtained his Ph.D. in clinical psychology from New York University.

Tatjana Zorcec, Ph.D., is a psychologist at the University Children's Hospital in Skopje, Macedonia. In 1993, she achieved her B.A. in psychology and in 2003 became a specialist in clinical psychology at the Medical

Faculty in Skopje. She also holds a master's degree and doctoral degree in medical sciences. In 2009, Dr. Zorcec was appointed as National Coordinator for Autism by the Macedonian Ministry of Health. In 2015, she became an associated professor at the Medical faculty. Dr. Zorcec gained additional education in several medical centers in Europe, the United States, and Australia. She is an active member in several national and international scientific projects, and author or co-author on 90 articles in scientific journals.